Epilepsy Handbook

Second Edition

By

LOUIS D. BOSHES, M.D.

Clinical Professor of Neurology
Director of the Consultation Clinic for Epilepsy
University of Illinois College of Medicine
Chicago, Illinois

and

FREDERIC A. GIBBS, M.D.

Professor of Neurology
Director of the Division of Electroencephalography
University of Illinois College of Medicine
Chicago, Illinois

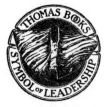

CHARLES C THOMAS • PUBLISHER

Springfield • Illinois • U.S.A.

Published and Distributed Throughout the World by
CHARLES C THOMAS • PUBLISHER
BANNERSTONE HOUSE
301–327 East Lawrence Avenue, Springfield, Illinois, U.S.A.
NATCHEZ PLANTATION HOUSE
735 North Atlantic Boulevard, Fort Lauderdale, Florida, U.S.A.

ISBN 0–398–02194–5

Library of Congress Catalog Card Number: 72-143730

First Edition, 1958

Second Edition, 1972

With THOMAS BOOKS *careful attention is given to all details of manufacturing and design. It is the Publisher's desire to present books that are satisfactory as to their physical qualities and artistic possibilities and appropriate for their particular use.* THOMAS BOOKS *will be true to those laws of quality that assure a good name and good will.*

Printed in the United States of America

BB-14

This book is dedicated to Dr. Eric Oldberg, Head of the Department of Neurology and Neurological Surgery at the University of Illinois College of Medicine. His kindness in providing funds and appointments for the Consultation Clinic for Epilepsy over a period of many years allowed it to flourish and expand even at the risk of unbalancing an otherwise perfectly balanced Department. Dr. Oldberg afforded us the opportunity to collect the data and allowed us the time to write this book, and we are grateful.

PREFACE TO THE SECOND EDITION

Since the first edition of this book was published thirteen years ago, much new information has developed concerning the diagnosis and treatment of convulsive and nonconvulsive forms of epilepsy. However, the text of the first edition was basically sound; it merely needed to be extended and supplemented, and in spite of Frederick Stamps' death in 1963, a revision of the Handbook seemed more desirable than publication of a new book under another title.

The purpose remains the same; this book is intended to be a compact, practical compendium of useful knowledge about epilepsy. Theory, discussion, and illustrations are held to a minimum. The bibliography includes references only to outstanding major works and to key articles on epilepsy. The current literature is now amply covered by *Epilepsy Abstracts*, published by the National Institute of Neurological Diseases and Blindness.

Although this is a little book, it was intended to be such from its inception. There are a number of excellent big books about epilepsy.[1,2,3,6] The biggest and the best, by William G. Lennox,[3] is full of scientific facts and also reports the weird ideas of ancient and not so ancient authorities; it is both instructive and entertaining. An admirable small book on epilepsy by Schmidt and Wilder[7] discusses the physiology and chemistry of epilepsy in more detail than we believed would be warranted in the present work. When Lennox reviewed the first edition of our little book, he gladdened our hearts by saying, "It contains no fat." We have tried to keep it that way.

Documentation for statements made here concerning the relationship between specific electroencephalographic patterns and types of clinical seizure can be found in the *Atlas of Electroencephalography*[8-10] or in more concise form in *Medical Electroencephalography*.[11]

vii

Because epilepsy can be caused by a great variety of diseases and conditions that injure the brain, an exhaustive book about epilepsy would necessarily include most of neurology and a large part of medicine. This book attempts to focus as sharply as possible on epilepsy. Important facts about this disorder become lost if they are included in the totality of what is known about diseases and disorders of the nervous system.

The busy doctor needs, and should have, answers to these highly pertinent questions: What is wrong with the patient? How can it be corrected? How can it be prevented? This book attempts to answer these questions as quickly, concisely, and clearly as the state of our present knowledge permits.

CONTENTS

EPILEPSY HANDBOOK

Chapter I

INTRODUCTION

Epilepsy is as common as diabetes and can masquerade in so many forms that any busy doctor will be treating it knowingly or unknowingly. If he attempts to read up on the subject by going to an older textbook, written before the advent of electroencephalography, or to recent texts that do not take into account the insights provided by electroencephalography, he will remain relatively unenlightened.

Hans Berger,[12,13] the father of electroencephalography, said, "The electroencephalogram is to the brain what the electrocardiogram is to the heart." But the electroencephalogram is even more; it shows clearly what otherwise is invisible. It reveals the disorder on which epilepsy is based, disordered regulation of the release of energy within the brain. It can show seizure activity even before it has manifested itself clinically. The electroencephalographic view of epilepsy does not replace the clinical view; these two views complement each other, just as the clinical and laboratory view complement each other in diabetes. They must be intelligently combined for the fullest understanding.

Epilepsy is evidence of an irritative reaction to some type of brain injury. It is nonspecific as regards etiology. The injury can be direct, as for example, from brain trauma or encephalitis; or it can be remote, for example, a transmitted genetic defect.[4] Some authors make a distinction between symptomatic epilepsy and genuine (essential or idiopathic) epilepsy. In the former, the seizures are a symptom of another disease or a consequence of structural damage to the brain; in the latter, they are supposed to be an expression of a brain disorder that has no structural basis and that is primary, i.e. not secondary to any

3

other disorder, injury, or disease process. This dichotomy disregards the fact that the essential lesion in epilepsy is a disorder of the intimate chemistry of cerebral neurons, resulting in an abnormal degree of neuronal instability; it is not based on structural changes. It is histologically invisible. Some day it will be diagnosable biochemically. Even with our present limited knowledge, however, the distinction between symptomatic and essential epilepsy is not useful. Cases of supposedly essential (or idiopathic) epilepsy are only those in which no assignable cause has been found.[5]

Chapter II

PAROXYSMAL CEREBRAL DYSRHYTHMIA

A small but significant fraction of the brain's total electrical output can be recorded in the electroencephalogram. The recording shows the fluctuating voltage production of cortical neurons in the outer convexity of the cerebral hemispheres. The activity of the neurons in the depths of the brain cannot be recorded. In sleep, however, certain deep-lying structures take over the control of the cortex, so that disorder in these deep (sleep) centers can be seen because their disorder is reflected in cortical disorder. Thus, sleep brings to the surface the activity of certain deep centers.

The flickering voltage production of the brain is much weaker and much faster than that of the heart. Its dominant rhythm, in healthy adults, is approximately ten cycles per second, and the voltage is measured in millionths of a volt. If one wishes to analogize the electroencephalogram and the electrocardiogram, the following two basic differences must be kept in mind: (a) the brain does not act like a unified organ, but like a population of small hearts with different interacting rhythms; (b) the pulsating electrical activity of the brain is not related to mechanical movement; it is related to the storage and release of nervous energy.

Energy conversion, release of energy, and limitation of energy release are important functions of the nerve cells of the brain. Sugar and oxygen are the basic fuels from which this nervous energy is obtained. Since part of the energy appears as electricity, the brain is in a real sense an electrochemical generator. The trouble with talking about electrical generators in the brain is that the generators with which most people are familiar are electromechanical, and of course, nothing of this sort is present in the brain. As in other tissue, voltage production in the brain

5

is chemical, and its regulation is chemical. A disorder of the brain's voltage production is evidence of disordered chemistry in cerebral neurons. In spite of much study, the chemical reactions that underlie the electrical activity of the brain are not clearly understood, and no one has pinpointed the chemical lesion or lesions responsible for epileptic seizures.

J. Hughlings Jackson[14] was the first to grasp the essential nature of epilepsy. It is due, he said, to a "discharging lesion." How right he was did not become apparent until the advent of electroencephalography made it possible to show the disordered release of energy within the brain. The epileptic's brain suddenly releases too much energy, and subsequently it releases too little. The fact that certain chemical substances are effective against one type of seizure discharge and not against others suggests that not one chemical lesion, but several, are responsible for the different varieties of epilepsy.

Lest at this point the reader becomes worried that he does not know enough about electricity, chemistry, or neurophysiology to proceed further, it may be helpful to remember that the respiratory center is a rhythmically acting brain center and one with which we have been familiar for hundreds of years. We do not know precisely what chemical processes underlie its rhythmic activity, and yet we make important clinical inferences from disturbances in respiratory rhythm. So also, while we are still ignorant about the chemical reactions responsible for the electrical activity of the brain, respiratory rhythm has told us a great deal about epilepsy. In most cases during a seizure and often in the interval between seizures, the brain of an epileptic can be shown to be in a dysrhythmic state. Electroencephalography has shown that epilepsy is in essence *paroxysmal cerebral dysrhythmia.*[15] As explained in the next chapter, in some cases of epilepsy a paroxysmal cerebral dysrhythmia cannot be demonstrated, but it is believed that abnormal electrical rhythms are present and invisible electroencephalographically, because they arise deep in the brain and do not reach the outer surface of the cerebral hemispheres, where they could be picked up with scalp electrodes.

Chapter III

TYPES OF EPILEPSY

Submaximal Seizures (Partial and Focal Epilepsy)

Epilepsy takes many forms depending on what part of the brain and how much of the brain is involved by the disordered energy release. If the discharge is confined to one part of the brain, it is *focal*. However, what starts as a focal discharge may spread and become generalized. The signs and symptoms that develop depend upon the functions subserved by the parts of the brain in which the disorder starts and to which it spreads. A focal seizure discharge can be associated with almost any of the symptoms or signs that the nervous system can produce, not only muscle contractions, but also hallucinations, rage, pain, and fever, to name but a few. The discharge can cause impairment of consciousness, complete unconsciousness, and in rare cases, heightened consciousness.

Clinical seizures that are not generalized tonic-clonic convulsions are submaximal, i.e. the discharge remains restricted to a part of the brain or is checked and limited temporally so that it does not develop maximal intensity. Even if the disorder involves the entire brain, a generalized convulsion does not necessarily occur, for the disturbance may be interrupted too quickly, i.e. checked in time. In petit mal epilepsy, for example, each single spike discharge is followed by a slow wave of depression. (See Fig. 11.) The spike and slow wave of petit mal epilepsy is commonly generalized, but it is submaximal in the *temporal* sense, and of course, a focal seizure is submaximal in the spatial sense. Examples of submaximal forms of epilepsy are the following: petit mal, petit mal variant, psychomotor, focal, Jacksonian, thalamic, and hypothalamic epilepsy.

7

Maximal Seizures (Generalized Tonic-Clonic Convulsions, Grand Mal Epilepsy)

If the discharges consist of a series of rapidly repeating fast waves or spikes (see Fig. 4) and if the patient is awake, the disturbance usually spreads widely, reaches the spinal cord and skeletal muscles, and manifests itself in the violent involuntary movement of a convulsive seizure. When the entire brain is involved, the seizure appears as a grand mal or generalized tonic-clonic convulsion.

The Age Factor

The form of epilepsy that develops is largely dependent on the age (the maturational state of the brain) at the time of injury (Fig. 1). The immature brain tends to react with a diffuse irritative response even when the injury is a localized one;

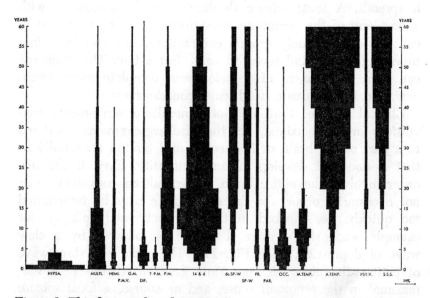

Figure 1. This figure is based on 19,350 consecutive cases with spike discharges, classified for age and type of discharge. The percentage incidence of each type in all age groups gives the age characteristic of that type of discharge. This is represented graphically as a segment of the total incidence of spikes at a given age; each segment is separated and moved so that

generalized paroxysmal dysrhythmias are far more common in children than in adults. The adult brain tends to show localized reactions to injury; focal dysrhythmias are more common in adults than in children. The part of the brain (and the particular maturational process) that at the time is undergoing maximal development is the one that is most vulnerable.[16] If focal epilepsy develops in infancy, it is usually in the occipital lobe; among school-age children it is usually in the midtemporal lobe, and among adults, in the anterior temporal lobe. Specific types of epilepsy will be considered in the order of the age at which they are most likely to develop. With increasing age, epilepsy tends to subside or to change to that form which is characteristic of the age the patient has attained.

Sleep

If the patient is in a natural or drug-induced sleep, the seizure discharge usually does not spread to the cord or motor nerves

---

it centers over corresponding segments showing the percentage incidence of that type of discharge in other age groups.

The contour of the area above each type of discharge shows the waxing and waning incidence of a particular pattern with age. The 20 percent calibration at the lower right margin allows the width of the column to be read as the percentage incidence of a particular type of discharge in a given age group; for example, 60 percent of persons with spikes, who are below one year of age, have hypsarhythmia; 65 percent of persons with spikes, who are 60 years of age or over, have anterior temporal spikes, and 50 percent of children between 10 and 15 years of age, who have spikes, have 14 and 6 per second positive spikes, etc. Abbreviations are as follows: HYPSA.—hypsarhythmia; MULTI.—multiple foci of spike seizure activity; HEMI.—spikes limited to one hemisphere; P.M.V.—discharge of the petit mal variant type; G.M.—discharge of the grand mal type; DIF.—diffuse nonspecific spike discharges; P P.M.—discharge of the pseudo petit mal type; P.M.—discharge of the petit mal type; 14 and 6—14 and 6 per second positive spikes; 6s.SP-W—6 per second spike-and-wave; SP-W—fronto-parietal spike-and-wave; FR.—spike focus in the frontal area; PAR.—spike focus in the parietal area; OCC.—spike focus in the occipital area: M.TEMP.—spike focus in the midtemporal area; A. TEMP.—spike focus in the anterior temporal area; PSY. V.—psychomotor variant type of discharge; S.S.S.—small sharp spikes. (From Gibbs, F.A., and Gibbs, E.L.: *Atlas of Electroencephalography*, Vol. 3, Addison-Wesley, 1964.)

but remains subclinical, i.e. unassociated with overt symptoms. However, if the patient is "aroused" during such a discharge, he may immediately show the outward manifestations of his seizure though he remains unconscious. The brain during sleep is de-efferented, like an automobile engine with the clutch disengaged. Arousal engages the "clutch," and the muscles respond to the streams of impulses that pour down the spinal cord from the brain.

Sleep is the ideal condition for recording seizure activity. Not only does the patient remain quiet during the seizure discharge, but there is also the additional advantage that seizure discharges in general are twice as likely to occur when the brain is "idling" in sleep as when it is awake (Fig. 2). Some types of seizure discharges are rarely seen in the waking state.

The electroencephalographic observation that seizure activity flares up during sleep is paralleled by the clinical observation

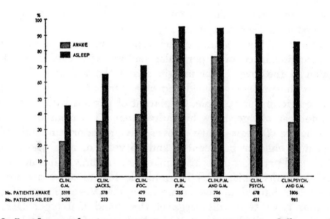

Figure. 2. Incidence of seizure activity among patients in different clinical diagnostic groups, studied awake and asleep.

This figure should be read as follows: 22 percent of 5,598 patients with clinical grand mal (and no other type of clinical seizure), whose electroencephalograms were recorded in the waking state, showed some type of seizure discharge, and 45.5 percent of 2,240 such patients, whose electroencephalograms were recorded during sleep, showed some type of seizure discharge. (From Gibbs, F.A., and Gibbs, E.L.: *Atlas of Electroencephalography*, vol. 2, Addison-Wesley, 1952.)

that seizures most commonly occur when the patient is going to sleep or is awakening. Some patients, particularly those with frequent petit mal or myoclonic seizures, have trouble getting dressed in the morning because, after arising, their seizures come in clusters and cease only when drowsiness is replaced by complete wakefulness.

Clinical and Electroencephalographic View

Electroencephalography is extremely useful in epilepsy, but it does not show everything. For example, a patient may have clinical epilepsy and yet have an entirely normal interseizure electroencephalogram. Epilepsy is a paroxysmal disorder, and even with sleep recordings, a paroxysm may not occur during an hour or more of recording. The clinical history provides a much longer "recording" than the electroencephalogram; it is a record of the patient's entire life, and it can record paroxysmal disturbances that occur only once in a lifetime.

A further limitation of the electroencephalogram is its inability to record discharges that are confined to the depths of the brain or to the mesial or inferior surfaces of the hemispheres. Thus, a patient may have clinical evidence of an epileptic focus, and yet disorder may not show in the electroencephalogram even during a clinical seizure. *Seizure discharges in the electroencephalogram are strongly suggestive of epilepsy, but negative findings (like a negative Wassermann reaction) are only presumptive evidence of normality.*

Negative electroencephalographic findings are especially common in patients with pure grand mal epilepsy (Fig. 2). Approximately one half of such patients are electroencephalographically normal or only slightly abnormal. This is not such a serious practical disadvantage as one might suppose, for in grand mal epilepsy the clinical manifestations are so obvious that laboratory verification is relatively unimportant. The electroencephalogram is most useful in cases with suspected or questionable epilepsy. In such cases, the detection of seizure discharges can clinch the diagnosis.

Like the clinical examination (and for that matter like any technique), electroencephalography has its blind spots. Full utilization of information from all sources leads to the most accurate diagnosis and to the selection of the most appropriate treatment. The clinical and electroencephalographic data should be combined and evaluated by a highly informed physician. If an electroencephalogram is not available or if it is technically unsatisfactory, the physician must proceed on the basis of his clinical evaluation and his general knowledge. From the clinical history alone it is possible to distinguish accurately a number of important entities. These are shown schematically in Figure 3a. When the electroencephalographic findings are used as the basis for classification, many of these same clinical entities can be distinguished, but some cannot (Fig. 3b). Certain entities that are not discernible clinically stand out sharply in the electro-encephalographic view.

>

Figure 3. (a) Viewed clinically, the universe of epilepsy reveals a variety of minor functional deviations from normal. The zones of minor deviation are surrounded and partially overlapped by a zone of extreme functional deviation, grand mal, which is undifferentiated except for febrile convulsions.

(b) Viewed in terms of interseizure electroencephalograms, the universe of epilepsy appears as a partially overlapping constellation of minor deviations from a field of apparent normality, which includes febrile convulsions and most of grand mal. The extreme deviation, grand mal, is nonevident except for a small area peripheral to petit mal and petit mal variant. Index marks (+) are provided to permit Fig. 3 (a) and (b) to be traced and superimposed, so that the degree of concordance between the clinical and electroencephalographic views can be estimated.

Some minor deviations can be seen clinically, but viewed electroencephalographically, they are more sharply defined and are seen to have subclinical forms (for example, petit mal and psychomotor epilepsy). Some minor deviations are easy to distinguish electroencephalographically and difficult to distinguish clinically (for example, petit mal variant). Pure grand mal and febrile convulsions can be clinically distinguished, but the interseizure electroencephalogram in these conditions seldom reveals any deviation from normal. (From Gibbs, F.A., and Gibbs, E.L.: *Atlas of Electroencephalography*, vol. 2, Addison-Wesley, 1952.)

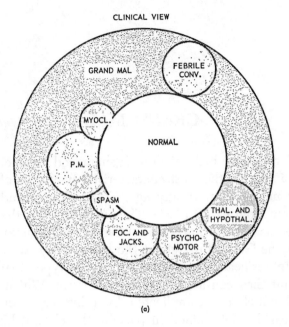

(a)

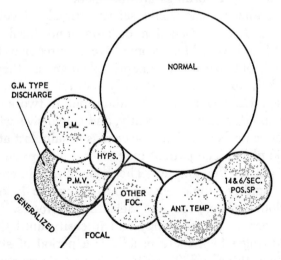

(b)

Chapter IV

GRAND MAL

Recurrent grand mal seizures (generalized tonic-clonic convulsions) are the most characteristic symptoms of epilepsy. They are not peculiar to any age. Their severity and duration vary widely from case to case. They indicate that the epileptic discharge has broken down spatial barriers and temporal checks and has gone "wild" throughout the brain. They can occur as a result of intensification and spread from any type of submaximal seizure, but they can also occur in pure form. Which cases are pure and which are complicated by other types of epileptic disorder can be determined in part by the clinical history, but more precisely from electroencephalographic studies, particularly when sleep recordings are included.

The generalized tonic-clonic seizure usually develops without warning. For a discussion of auras and focal signs, see Chapters XI and XIV. Major convulsive seizures may be diurnal or nocturnal, but like other epileptic phenomena, they are particularly likely to occur in the early morning, at the end of a night's sleep. They commonly last about one to two minutes, but frequency and duration vary greatly, and convulsive seizures may occur in series for hours. Consciousness is usually lost at the onset of the tonic phase. The patient may utter a high-pitched cry and slump or fall to the ground. The generalized intense spasms start with rigidity (tonic phase) and change to jerking movements (clonic phase) as the seizure progresses. The jerks gradually decrease in frequency and intensity until they finally cease, following which there usually is a period of stupor with stertorous breathing and flaccidity. This postseizure stupor varies in duration; usually it is longer after a prolonged and severe seizure than after a mild and short one. As the stupor wears off,

14

the patient may lapse into sleep or occasionally into a period of excitement. As a rule he is amnestic for the entire episode, but usually he knows that he has had a seizure. Disruption of normal autonomic function may be profound. If the tongue and lips are bitten, saliva may be blood-tinged. Jaw or shoulder joints may be dislocated, and micturation and, less commonly, defecation may occur during severe attacks. Even without these complications, there are usually unpleasant after-effects, for example, muscular soreness or weakness, headache, vomiting, malaise, or depression.

Grand Mal Type of Discharges

The characteristic electroencephalographic changes that occur in immediate temporal association with a generalized tonic-clonic (grand mal) seizure (Fig. 4) consist of an abrupt decrease in voltage followed by a generalized rapid build-up of spikes or fast activity. These increase in amplitude and decrease in frequency throughout the tonic phase. Slow waves interspersed with bursts of spikes are characteristic of the clonic phase. The bursts of

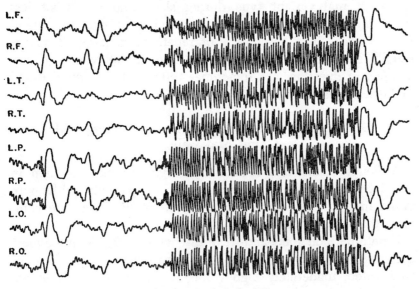

Figure 4. Grand mal.

spikes usually coincide with the jerks of the clonic phase. When the seizure discharge terminates and the clonic phase ends, very slow activity develops in the postseizure phase, but if the seizure has been very severe and prolonged, flattening may occur. With recovery, waves of increasing frequency appear until gradually the patient's characteristic preictal activity is restored. Commonly, however, it is interspersed with slow waves that may take hours or days to disappear. Commonly, also, preictal activity does not appear until after a fairly long period of normal sleep.

The grand mal type of discharge develops so rapidly and generalizes so completely that in the waking state it is rarely seen except in association with a major tonic-clonic convulsion. The convulsion produces such a great amount of muscle potential and movement artifact that the electroencephalogram is obliterated. Clearly identifiable grand mal discharges are rarely recorded except during sleep or during status epilepticus. In sleep, as previously stated, intense discharges can occur without spreading to the spinal cord and without causing muscular activity or movement artifacts. Subclinical grand mal discharges are most commonly observed among patients with epilepsy of the petit mal variant type during sleep and somewhat less commonly among patients with clinical petit mal and grand mal seizures. Short discharges of repetitive generalized spikes, usually occurring during sleep and approximately one or two seconds in duration, are sometimes referred to as *larval* grand mal discharges.

Other Types of Seizure Activity Correlating with Grand Mal Epilepsy

Although grand mal seizure discharges are not common in the interseizure electroencephalogram of patients with pure grand mal epilepsy, certain other types of discharge are common; they are as follows:

Fronto-parietal spike-and-wave discharges (Fig. 5) are almost exclusively an adult abnormality. They occur in the form of an isolated, moderately high voltage spike-and-wave discharge with a duration of one fourth to one third of a second. The

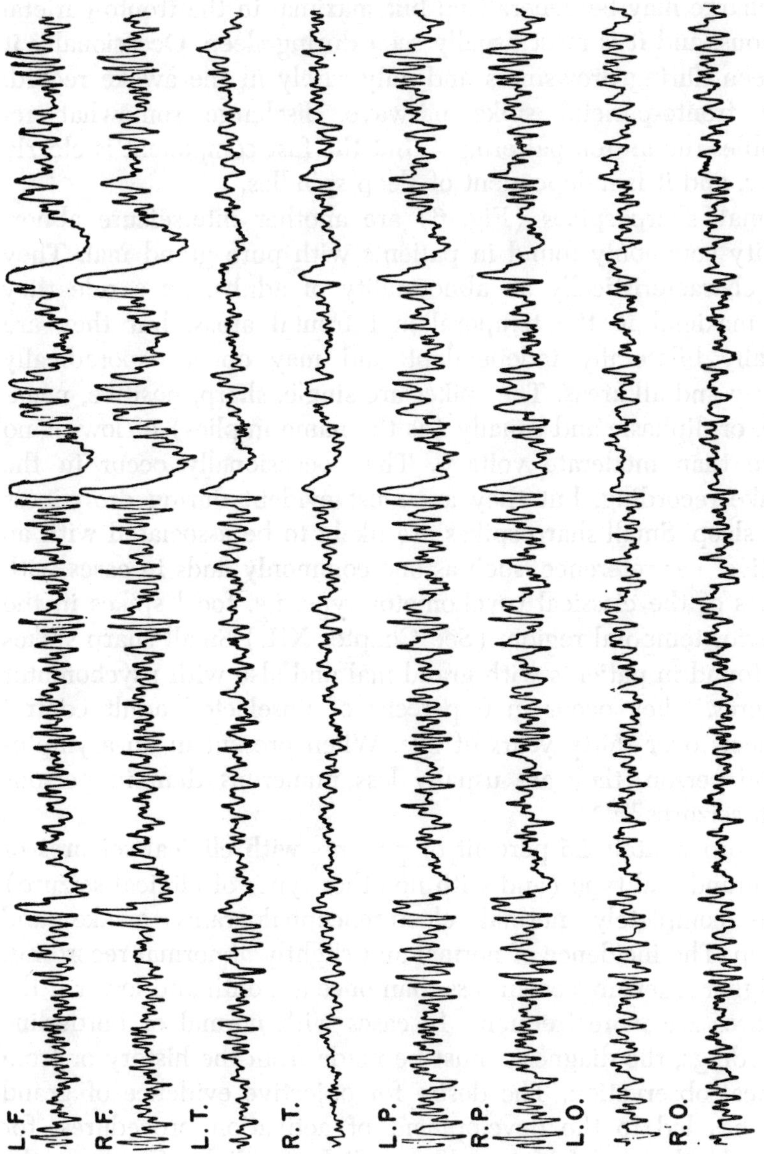

Figure 5. Fronto-parietal spike-and-wave activity.

discharge may be generalized but maximal in the fronto-parietal regions, and it is most usually seen during sleep. Occasionally it is seen during drowsiness and only rarely in the awake record. The fronto-parietal spike-and-wave discharge somewhat resembles the mitten pattern,[10,11] but the fast component is clearly spiky, and it is independent of sleep spindles.

Small sharp spikes (Fig. 6) are another interseizure abnormality commonly found in patients with pure grand mal. They are characteristically an abnormality of adults. As a rule they are maximal in the temporal and frontal areas, but they are usually bilaterally independent and may appear sporadically in any and all areas. The spikes are single, sharp, positive, negative, or diphasic and usually (as the name implies) of low or no more than moderate voltage. They occasionally occur in the awake recording, but they are most evident during drowsiness and sleep. Small sharp spikes are likely to be associated with an "active" ear reference, such as one commonly finds in cases with spikes of the classical psychomotor type, i.e. focal spikes in the anterior temporal region. (See Chapter XII.) Small sharp spikes are found in patients with grand mal and also with psychomotor seizures. They occur in 6 percent of unselected adult control subjects over thirty years of age. When present in an asymptomatic person, they are usually less numerous than in persons with seizures.[17,18]

Approximately 25 percent of patients with clinical seizures of the grand mal type (and with no other types of clinical seizure) have completely normal electroencephalograms awake and asleep. The incidence of normal and slightly abnormal recordings is higher if seizures occur less than once a month and lower if the seizures are more frequent. In cases with normal or borderline recordings, the diagnosis must be made from the history or from clinical observation. The desire for objective evidence of grand mal has led to the development of activation procedures, for example, the use of Metrazol® and flickering light. However, the overlap between epileptics and normal controls is so great that these activation procedures are not of great practical value.[19-22] From a practical point of view, in ordinary practice, objective

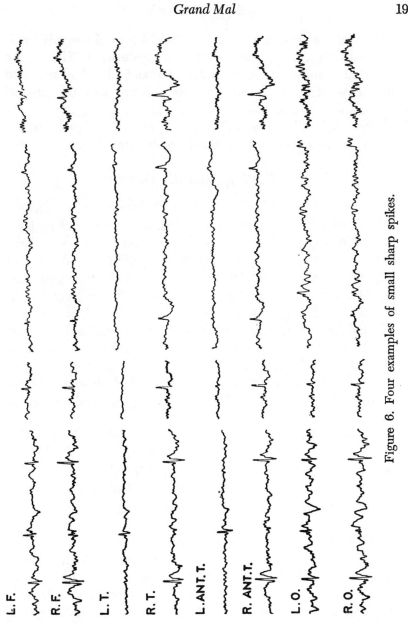

L.F.

R.F.

L.T.

R.T.

L. ANT. T.

R. ANT. T.

L.O.

R.O.

Figure 6. Four examples of small sharp spikes.

evidence of epilepsy in a patient with a history of convulsions is not usually necessary. (See section on hysteria, p. 81.) If the patient, his family, or observers report that he has had repeated convulsions, if in other respects the history and the clinical examinations are noncontributory, a reasonable diagnosis would be "grand mal epilepsy" even if the interseizure electroencephalogram both awake and asleep shows no abnormalities.

Complicating Epileptic Disorder

When carefully studied electroencephalographically, particularly when a sleep recording is included, the majority of patients with supposedly pure grand mal epilepsy can be shown to have additional types of epileptic disorder. Depending on the age of the patient, hypsarhythmia, petit mal variant, and petit mal types of discharges as well as fourteen and six per second positive spikes and single or multiple foci of spike seizure activity are found in patients with supposedly pure grand mal epilepsy. These types of disorders are dealt with in detail in later sections.

Nonparoxysmal abnormality, for example, an excess of fast or slow activity, may also be present. Marked slowing is common in patients who have had frequent, prolonged, or recent seizures.

In some cases careful review of the history indicates that types of seizure discharge (other than grand mal) which were supposedly subclinical have in fact produced symptoms that were either previously overlooked or were believed to be nonepileptic. In many cases, however, the complicating types of seizure discharge are actually subclinical.

The prognosis varies with the cause, frequency, and severity of grand mal attacks, the type and degree of electroencephalographic abnormality, and the age of the patient. In general, seizures of unknown cause that are infrequent and relatively mild have a good prognosis with proper treatment. Approximately 85 percent of cases with pure grand mal seizures can be controlled with present anticonvulsant drugs. The chances of eventual complete cessation of seizures with normalization of the electroencephalogram varies with the initial type of abnormality and with the age of onset. (See sections dealing with types of seizure discharge and with age.)

The etiology of grand mal seizures (and seizures of all types) is non-specific and usually unknown. They can be caused by anything that injures the brain, for example, trauma, lack of oxygen, vascular disease, encephalitis,[23] toxins of many types, neoplasms,[25] fungus diseases,[24,26,27] and metabolic disorders. The etiologic diagnosis is of great importance (see p. 87), but anticonvulsant medication can reduce symptoms regardless of the cause of the epilepsy. Hereditary factors play a role in grand mal seizures as they do in other types of epilepsy. As will be pointed out in Chapter VI, a genetic factor is especially important in febrile convulsions.

Chapter V

INFANTILE SPASMS (WEST'S SYNDROME) AND HYPSARHYTHMIA

Infants and young children with a history of frequent, brief spasms or quivering spells (sometimes called "twitch," "nodding," or "salaam" seizures, and occasionally termed "massive myoclonia") usually have an exceedingly abnormal interseizure electroencephalogram of a special type. The abnormal pattern is referred to as *hypsarhythmia*.*[28] The chief long-term hazard faced by patients with this pattern is not epilepsy, bad as this may be, but mental retardation. No other epileptic pattern is so commonly associated with impaired intellectual development. An infant or young child who initially has a single spike focus or multiple foci of spike seizure activity is threatened with hypsarhythmia if the number and voltage of the spikes steadily increases. This abnormality can develop rapidly or slowly. When fully developed, normal cortical activity disappears and is replaced by random high voltage slow waves and spikes in all areas. The spikes vary from moment to moment both in duration and location and may be single or multiple (Fig. 7). At times they seem to come from a single focus, but a few seconds later they can be seen to originate from multiple foci. Occasionally the spike discharge is generalized, but it never becomes synchronized and highly organized like the spike-and-wave of petit mal variant (Fig. 10) or of true petit mal (Fig. 11). Hypsarhythmia is present in the interval between clinically evident spasms, and it usually shows both awake and asleep. However, when it is minimal, it shows in the sleep recording only. In severe cases the discharge is almost continuous, but in

---

* The prefix *hypsi* means mountainous or lofty. The word *hypsarhythmia* is spelled with one *r* in the interest of simplicity.

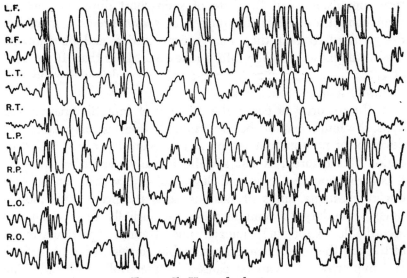

Figure 7. Hypsarhythmia.

the severest cases it is interrupted by periods of flattening. If the case is one that is responding to treatment or if the disorder is subsiding, as it commonly does with increasing age, the high voltage discharges are interrupted by normal activity. When the hypsarhythmia clears up, the child may be left with multiple foci of spike seizure activity, a single spike focus, or a normal electroencephalogram.

This disorder is most likely to occur in the first year of life. It is rare after the age of three; it is extremely uncommon after the age of ten. As in most types of epilepsy, males are more often affected than females. The seizures are characterized by one or more of the following: a cry accompanied by sudden flexion of the head, rolling of the eyes, upward flinging of the arms, flexion of the thighs, or quivering of the entire body. Each seizure lasts about a second; they commonly occur in showers, but the movements are not rhythmically repeated as in the classical petit mal seizure. Though abrupt and brief, the attacks are not as short nor as lightning-like as *myoclonic* seizures. Commonly they occur when the patient is awake, and they also occur during sleep. They could be considered miniature convulsions, but they are of such short duration that the term *convulsion* seems inappropriate; *spasm* seems a more apt designation. At first they may escape notice and occasionally are misdiagnosed as colic, Moro reflex, etc. Less than 10 percent of cases have generalized, tonic-clonic convulsions (grand mal seizures) as a complication.

In the majority of cases, the etiology of infantile spasms and hypsarhythmia cannot be determined. Spasms may suddenly develop for no apparent reason in a previously normal infant or child. This disorder is not specific for any particular etiology; it is a reaction to a type and degree of injury that can be produced by many kinds of noxious agents. Encephalitis (sometimes secondary to immunization but usually due to an unidentifiable pathogen), anoxia, and trauma (particularly at birth) are the most common assignable causes. Infantile spasms and hypsarhythmia can be caused by metabolic and endocrine disorders, notably phenylketonuria, pyridoxine deficiency, hypocalcemia, and hypoglycemia. Of course, when the primary etiology can be found, it should be remedied if possible. Hypsarhythmia may be associated with severe neurological defects, with cerebral palsy, with developmental defects, such as microcephaly, with mongolism, and occasionally, with cerebral atrophy. No cases with tumor has been reported. Hereditary factors do not seem to be of great importance in this condition.

Early diagnosis and intensive treatment with ACTH (see p. 135) are urgent, for even though spasms may be controlled or eliminated and the EEG normalized, intellectual defects occur quickly and are likely to be permanent. The prognosis in infantile spasms and hypsarhythmia is worse than in almost any other common form of epilepsy. When not treated with ACTH 11 percent of patients die before the third year of life and approximately 80 percent of those that live are severely retarded. The spasms and hypsarhythmia tend to subside by the third or fourth year, but generalized convulsions, often associated with multiple spike foci in the electroencephalogram, may continue for many years. Severe neuromuscular and intellectual impairment is the chief long-term hazard.

Chapter VI

FEBRILE CONVULSIONS

Febrile convulsions might not seem to be a logical diagnostic entity. However, about 3 percent of children below five years of age have convulsions with febrile illnesses and not in afebrile periods. This is a specific but relatively benign form of epilepsy, which, as a rule, clears up spontaneously with increasing age and is not followed by any other type of disorder.[29,30] This chapter dealing with it may seem inappropriately located, falling as it does between chapters which deal with two of the most severe forms of epilepsy, namely, hypsarhythmia and petit mal variant. However, since true febrile convulsions occur in infants and young children, this chapter is presented at this juncture in accordance with the principle adhered to in this book; the various types of epileptic disorders are considered in the order in which they make their appearance in the course of growth and development.

Febrile convulsions are the result of a specific abnormality, a low convulsive threshhold for increased body temperature. Although one might assume that these convulsions are a form of "symptomatic" epilepsy, because of the precipitating role of the febrile illness, the familial incidence of febrile convulsions is high, higher in fact than in most other types of epilepsy (Fig. 8). What is inherited is not epilepsy in general but a specific and limited defect which is associated with a strong tendency to spontaneous recovery.[29,30]

The following are the significant diagnostic criteria: convulsions occurring only with febrile illnesses, usually soon after the onset of the illness and at the height of the fever (although it may not be especially high). The seizures are generalized and brief, usually under ten minutes, and there are no sequelae. A child may experience only one febrile convulsion, but as a rule true febrile convulsions occur repeatedly with febrile illnesses one to four times a year, depending on the exposure to infection. Prolonged or focal seizures, afebrile convulsions, or convulsions occurring with fever in a child more than five years of age raise questions as to the correctness of the diagnosis.[30]

The electroencephalogram is of special value in the diagnosis of febrile convulsions. If recorded during the febrile period, slowing may be present, but if the case is truly one of uncom-

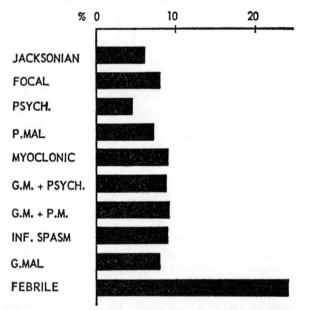

Figure 8. Incidence of a positive family history of epilepsy in different types of clinical epilepsy. A history of seizures in parents, siblings, grandparents, aunts, or uncles was considered a positive family history. (More distant relatives were not included.)

For the purpose of the analysis, no distinction was made between cases in which several relatives had seizures and cases in which only one was affected. Abbreviations are as follows: INF. SPASM—infantile spasms; MYOCLONIC—myoclonic seizures; FOCAL—focal convulsions; JACKSONIAN—Jacksonian seizures; G.M. and PSYCH.—grand mal and psychomotor seizures; G.M. and P.M.—grand mal and petit mal; P.MAL—clinical petit mal with no other type of clinical seizure; G.MAL—clinical grand mal with no other type of clinical seizure; PSYCH.—psychomotor seizures; FEBRILE—febrile convulsions. (From Gibbs, F.A., and Gibbs, E.L.: *Atlas of Electroencephalography*, vol. 2, Addison-Wesley, Reading, Mass., 1952.)

plicated febrile convulsions, the interseizure routine electroencephalogram (taken when the child has been afebrile for several days), will be normal awake and asleep. A slight exception to the foregoing statement is dealt with in the next section.

Pseudo Petit Mal Discharge

A rare electroencephalographic pattern which is encountered in some normal children and some children with febrile convulsions has been termed *pseudo petit mal* (Fig. 9). It correlates with febrile convulsions and with no other disorder. It occurs among infants and young children and is seen during drowsiness and very light sleep. It consists of irregular high voltage diffuse three to four per second slow waves, similar to the normal slow waves of drowsiness in young children, but it is interspersed with a few random spikes, usually maximal in the parietal areas. Unlike the classical, regular three per second spike-and-wave discharge of the petit mal type, it does not occur in the awake recording, nor in deep sleep. Other distinguishing features are these: it is not precipitated by hyperventilation, and it is never associated with clinical petit mal seizures. Pseudo petit mal can be properly regarded as a mild paroxysmal dysrhythmia, which almost always disappears with age and which is usually asymptomatic, but which in some cases is associated with febrile convulsions. Rarely other more serious abnormalities replace it; repeat recordings are advisable at yearly intervals to make sure that the electroencephalogram has become entirely normal.

Febrile convulsions, with their good prognosis, high hereditary factor, and usual absence of serious electroencephalographic abnormality, are not always recognized as a distinct entity; they are easily confused with more serious syndromes. A patient should not be diagnosed as having febrile convulsions merely because a convulsion has occurred in association with fever. The convulsion may be a sign of encephalitis or of a septic infarct. When a convulsion occurs with fever at an early age, the electroencephalogram is helpful for making an accurate differential diagnosis.[30] If marked diffuse or focal slowing persists in the recording one to two weeks after the temperature is normal or

Epilepsy Handbook

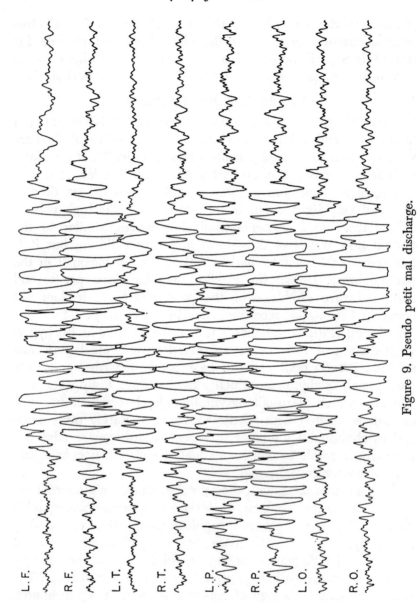

L.F.

R.F.

L.T.

R.T.

L.P.

R.P.

L.O.

R.O.

Figure 9. Pseudo petit mal discharge.

if a repeat recording after one month or more reveals slowing or spiking, the case is not one of uncomplicated febrile convulsions but more probably one of convulsions secondary to encephalitis. Approximately 50 percent of the patients who had encephalitis with convulsions in the acute phase of their illness have abnormal follow-up electroencephalograms. (See Chapter XVII.) A normal follow-up recording after a febrile convulsion has prognostic value; it gives some assurance that afebrile seizures will not occur at a later date.

Other conditions must be differentiated from simple febrile convulsions. Occasionally, cases of epilepsy are encountered where the fever itself is a consequence of an autonomic seizure discharge, or the case may be one in which the body temperature is elevated secondary to a violent convulsion. Convulsions occasionally result from the treatment of the infection rather than from the fever itself, for instance as a result of excessive hydration or from large doses of certain drugs. Some patients may have a local onset to their seizures and may remain comatose during a prolonged recovery period. This is sometimes called "infantile hemiplegia" and may be the result of cerebral venous thrombosis. In such cases focal electroencephalographic abnormalities and seizures often persist, and it is obvious that the case cannot be properly classified as true febrile convulsions.

The etiology of febrile convulsions seems to be chiefly an inherited defect. Since this disorder is so inheritable, it is fortunate that it is so benign. Because convulsions are usually mild and relatively infrequent, treatment is not imperative. The use of anticonvulsant medication only during the febrile periods is somewhat impractical. In most instances the fever shoots up, and the child has a convulsion before medicine can be administered. However, it is not unreasonable to give the child phenobarbital or other anticonvulsant medication along with aspirin when the temperature elevation is first noted and for a few days following the onset of the fever. If prolonged convulsions occur or if they come close together, the child should be placed on maintenance anticonvulsant medication until the age of five or six.

Chapter VII

PETIT MAL VARIANT EPILEPSY AND AKINETIC SEIZURES

Petit mal variant is essentially an electroencephalographic diagnosis because the characteristic discharge, shown in Figure 10, even when prolonged, is not usually accompanied by immediate clinical manifestations.[31,32] The pattern consists of generalized, high voltage, approximately two per second spike-and-wave discharges. The spikes are somewhat blunt, and the slow waves have a relatively fast rise and a slower fall often with several notches or ripples on the descending slope. As a rule they are maximal in the frontal and parietal regions, but occasionally they predominate in one area or one hemisphere. They can appear in the awake or in the sleep recording, but are usually most numerous during drowsiness and sleep. The spikes are often multiple, especially during sleep, and bursts of high voltage multiple spikes are common. A grand mal type of discharge usually accompanies the patient's clinical seizures.

The petit mal variant type of discharge is most common among young children, but the abnormality is occasionally found among adults. Usually the chief complaint is of severe and frequent generalized convulsions; brief attacks of impaired consciousness occur in some cases. The latter are associated with one or more of the following: nodding of the head, sudden loss of motion or posture with varying degrees of muscular relaxation. This type of seizure has been called "akinetic," "atonic," "astatic," or "drop seizures."[3] They often cause the patient to pitch forward or backward; he often goes down with a crash, and head injuries frequently result from this type of seizure unless the patient wears a helmet or some other type of protective head gear. These akinetic seizures may occur hundreds of times a day. As previously stated, the discharge that

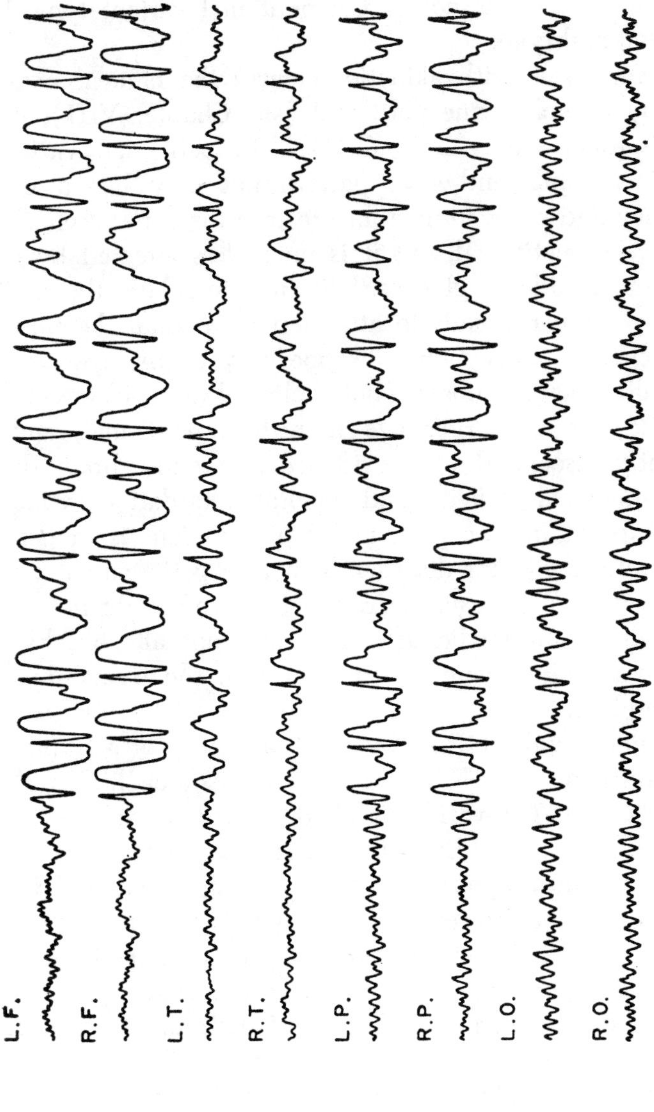

Figure 10. Petit mal variant discharge.

accompanies them is not of the petit mal variant type, but of the grand mal type.

In some cases with akinetic seizures the clinical manifestation may resemble true petit mal (see Chapter VIII), but the two disorders are entirely distinct. In petit mal variant the interseizure spike-and-wave pattern not only has a different frequency and wave form from the true three per second spike-and-wave of petit mal, but it is much less affected by change in carbon dioxide or glucose.[31] Strange to relate, the petit mal variant pattern responds to attention more than the pure petit mal discharge; it commonly disappears when the eyes are open. It usually has its onset (both clinical and electroencephalographic) at an earlier age than true petit mal, and it is frequently associated with evidence of organic brain damage, i.e. neurological deficits and mental retardation, which are usually absent in true petit mal.[32] The variant is in general a much more malignant disorder than true petit mal; major convulsive seizures are usually frequent and often do not respond to anticonvulsant medication. They are not affected by drugs that are specific for pure petit mal (i.e. the oxazolidines and succinimides).

In patients with petit mal variant, a history of a traumatic or anoxic birth or encephalitis in infancy is much higher than in pure petit mal. The variant is almost never caused by a tumor. In this condition, hereditary factors are not especially important.

Although the prognosis is not as bad as in cases of infantile spasm, the outlook in general is not good; severe uncontrollable convulsions usually continue in spite of treatment, and intellectual deficits are a common end result. Many patients with this abnormality have to be institutionalized. With increasing age the petit mal variant pattern usually clears up, but the electroencephalogram remains abnormal because multiple foci of spike seizure activity develop, and clinical seizures usually continue.

Chapter VIII

PETIT MAL

The term *petit mal* is now used in a restricted sense. Before the advent of electroencephalography, it was commonly applied in a roughly quantitative manner to any type of mild seizure. True petit mal seizures are characterized clinically by brief (usually 5–30 sec in duration), frequent (5–100 or more per day) attacks of impaired consciousness (absences), rarely associated with any sensation or aura.[3] They manifest themselves clinically by one or more of the following: rhythmic blinking of the eyes, nodding of the head, jerking of the arms, staring, and sudden loss of posture. In some cases the patient has urinary incontinence, but often the only clue that the patient has to the fact that he has experienced a seizure is an awareness that time has passed unaccountably. Such seizures are characteristically a disorder of childhood and adolescence; they tend to clear up with increasing age.

This type of seizure was formerly referred to as pyknolepsy in the belief that it is not true epilepsy. More recently it has been called centrencephalic epilepsy on the assumption that it originates in the thalamus,[33] an assumption that has been shown to be erroneous.[34-36,39]

Attention tends to prevent petit mal seizures, but relaxation and drowsiness tend to increase them. Usually they are most numerous shortly after awakening; sometimes they occur so close together that the patient has difficulty getting dressed. They can in some cases be interrupted by sensory stimulation, and in some cases they are precipitated by embarrassment. When prolonged and occurring in close succession, they can constitute a *petit mal status,* a condition which in itself is not dangerous, but unless identified electroencephalographically, it is likely to be misinterpreted as stupor due to some life threatening disturbance.

Petit mal epilepsy is associated with a specific and characteristic pattern in the electroencephalogram,[37] namely, high voltage spike-and-wave discharges, which repeat rhythmically with a frequency of approximately three per second (Fig. 11). The discharge is usually generalized, and in the youngest age group, maximal in the occipital areas, but in older children and adults the highest voltages are usually recorded from the frontal and parietal areas. Occasionally other areas are maximally involved, and rarely is the discharge lateralized or focal. The bursts are brief during subclinical discharges, and more prolonged (usually in excess of 3 sec) during a clinical seizure. They are usually faster at the outset and become slower as the discharge continues. Sometimes bursts of three per second slow waves without spikes are present, especially in the occipital areas, and independent focal spikes are not an unusual complication. For some unknown reason, petit mal seizures and psychomotor seizures (with an anterior temporal spike focus) are almost never associated. In cases of petit mal, the interparoxysmal

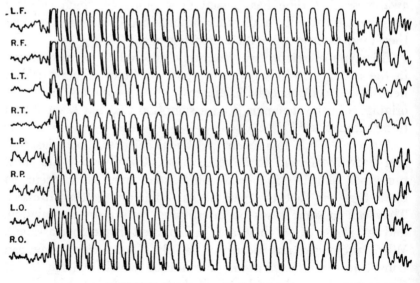

Figure 11. Petit mal discharge.

recording, as a rule, is normal or slightly slow. Petit mal discharges and sometimes clinical seizures can be precipitated by hypoglycemia, by hyperventilation (hypocapnia), and readily by anoxia.[31] Having the patient take one hundred or more deep breaths in a period of two to three minutes (hyperventilation) may reveal seizure activity that was not present in the awake recording. However, petit mal discharges are rarely obtained with hyperventilation, if they are not evident during sleep. Some patients with petit mal are sensitive to photic stimulation and develop seizure discharges or may even develop clinical seizures when confronted with a bright flickering light.[38]

Discharges of the petit mal type are commonly seen both awake and asleep, but they are more numerous during sleep than in the awake recording, and in some cases they show only in sleep. During sleep their form is more irregular than in the awake recording, and they often appear to be focal, but the foci are usually multiple and shifting. Sleep intensifies any grand mal component that is present.

Petit mal seizures are rare in children below two years of age; they are most common between five and nineteen years of age. They tend to disappear with increasing age and are relatively rare in adults. (See Fig. 1.) However, in some cases, when clinical seizures have ceased, poorly organized bursts of spike-and-wave discharges persist in the electroencephalogram. Cases complicated by generalized tonic-clonic seizures (grand mal) tend to have a later age of onset than cases with petit mal only, but convulsive seizures can precede or follow the onset of petit mal seizures. Among patients with grand mal, multiple spikes or groups of spikes are commonly mixed with the petit mal discharges (especially in sleep recordings). These are referred to as a *grand mal component*. In cases with a strong grand mal component, the prognosis must be guarded, for grand mal seizures are likely to develop later if they have not done so already, and patients with a mixture of grand mal and petit mal are likely to be therapeutic problems. (See page 125.) However, less than one half of the patients with childhood petit mal go on to develop grand mal seizures. The petit mal type of discharge, unlike all other forms of epilepsy, except the six per second spike-and-wave discharge, is more common among females than among males.

⋆The intelligence of patients with petit mal epilepsy is usually in the median range or higher, and personality disorders are rare. Evidence of brain damage is also rare, in contrast to the high incidence of brain damage among patients with petit mal variant discharges. Other reports to the contrary not with-standing,[39,40] the hereditary factor in petit mal epilepsy seems to be no greater than in most types of epilepsy, and it is less than in febrile convulsions (Fig. 8). Encephalitis is the most common presumptive etiology, but in the majority of cases no cause can be found. Trauma, birth injury, and tumors rarely cause petit mal epilepsy, nor do chronic progressive diseases; this disorder is unrelated to brain anomalies or dysplasias.

Chapter IX

MYOCLONIC EPILEPSY

Myoclonic seizures are characterized clinically by a single, sudden, violent jerk of the head and neck, the arms, and sometimes the trunk and legs, without observable loss of consciousness. Attacks tend to diminish with advancing age,[3] but less so than in cases of petit mal epilepsy. The prognosis is generally good. They are usually associated with short bursts of generalized high voltage spike-and-wave complexes with multiple spikes in the electroencephalogram.[9] When the discharge is accompanied by a clinically evident myoclonic jerk, it is likely (as might be expected) to be complicated by movement artifacts.

In cases with mild myoclonic seizures, only the head, neck, shoulders, or arms may be involved, and the movement may be either extension or flexion. The patient is sometimes thrown off balance if standing or catapulted from his chair if seated. A single seizure lasts only one or two seconds, and consciousness is not noticeably impaired; usually the patient is entirely lucid and is annoyed or embarrassed by his explosive, uncontrollable movements. These seizures usually occur in showers of four or five with an interval of three to six seconds between; their frequency varies greatly. They are particularly likely to occur on awakening or on going to sleep. Some patients find it almost impossible to get dressed in the morning because of a storm of myoclonic seizures.

Almost two thirds (64%) of the patients with myoclonic epilepsy have grand mal convulsions, and 21 percent have clinical petit mal seizures; less than 2 percent have psychomotor seizures.[9] Infantile spasms with hypsarhythmia (see Chapter V) are sometimes referred to as "massive myoclonia."[3]

37

Myoclonic epilepsy has no specific etiology. Neurological, psychiatric, and mental defects are not common in pure cases. Trauma and encephalitis are the most usual presumptive causes. Hereditary factors are about as common as in petit mal epilepsy (Fig. 8), but less important than in cases with febrile convulsions.

Myoclonus is distinct from myoclonic epilepsy.[3] It (myoclonus) is characterized by irregular, frequent involuntary muscular jerks which may migrate from one part of the body to another. It occurs as an outstanding symptom in a number of rare progressive cerebral degenerative diseases, such as inclusion body encephalitis, Unverricht-Lundborg disease, Jakob-Creutzfeldt's disease, and certain cerebrovascular degenerative diseases. Generalized and focal seizures may also be present in these cases. As the disorder progresses, the electroencephalogram awake and asleep commonly shows increasing amounts of diffuse high voltage slow activity mixed with spikes, occurring periodically and followed by flattening.

Some cases which closely resemble myoclonic epilepsy in their clinical manifestations have normal electroencephalograms awake and asleep during the seizure-free interval. In such cases the electroencephalogram may remain normal even during the clinically evident myoclonic attacks. Such cases are presumably the result of a discharge in lower centers that do not project to the cortex. Patients with hemiballismus have jerking which is confined to one side of the body; in this condition the electroencephalogram is usually normal. The sudden jerks of the legs or other parts of the body that are common in normal persons as they doze off to sleep are unassociated with electroencephalographic abnormality and are apparently unrelated to epilepsy or to any other type of central nervous dysfunction. Myoclonic jerks in patients with myoclonic epilepsy are often induced by sudden unexpected stimuli (see Chapter XIII), but they are distinguishable from the normal startle response by their excessive forcefulness and by the fact that they also occur spontaneously without startling stimuli. Tics, habit spasms, or chorea sometimes superficially resemble myoclonic epilepsy, but differ widely in causation and treatment. Although the electroencephalogram may be abnormal in some patients with these last mentioned conditions (see pp. 69, 70), they are not associated with the generalized multiple spike and slow wave discharges that usually occur in myoclonic epilepsy.

The so-called photomyoclonic response is distinct from myoclonic epilepsy. It is associated with a run of high voltage rhythmic "spikes" in the frontal areas and clinically with muscular jerking mainly in the periorbital and facial regions. It is precipitated by photic stimulation, is especially common in tense, normal subjects, and has almost no clinical significance.

Chapter X

DIENCEPHALIC (THALAMIC AND HYPOTHALAMIC) EPILEPSY

For many years authorities have recognized that seizure activity in the central gray masses of the brain can give rise to episodic symptoms. Cases have been described where one or more of the following, headaches, dizzy spells, attacks of nausea and vomiting, sweating, palpitation of the heart, disturbances of respiration, and rage, were said to be "epileptic equivalents."[3] Because such symptoms are so common and are more often than not on a nonepileptic basis, a clinical diagnosis of epilepsy could be made with confidence only when a sudden flare-up of such nonspecific symptoms was followed by unconsciousness or convulsive movements. Nonconvulsive symptoms occurring at the start of a convulsion can be properly classified as *auras* (see p. 64), but they can occur alone and be on an epileptic basis.

Electroencephalographic studies of patients with auras, partial seizures, and equivalents, which suggested a discharge originating in the diencephalon (thalamus or hypothalamus) were found to have a high incidence of a distinctive sleep pattern, namely, fourteen and six per second positive spikes.[41] This pattern (Fig. 12) was found also in many persons with sensory seizures and atypical spells, for example, attacks of numbness, pain, tingling, or formication in the arms, legs, or trunk. Patients with episodic illusion were also found to have positive spiking during sleep. Some reported one or more of the following strange experiences: "All of a sudden everything becomes very bright," ". . . very dim," ". . . very loud," ". . . very quiet," ". . . very big,"* ". . . very small."† Another type of episodic illusion reported by

---

* macropsia
† micropsia

40

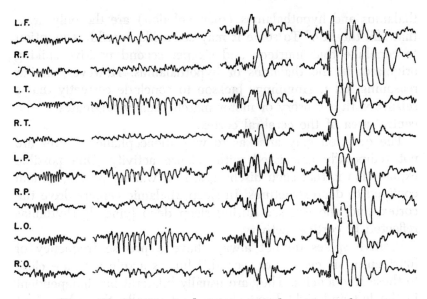

Figure 12. Fourteen and six per second positive spikes.

patients with fourteen and six per second positive spikes was the feeling that everything was going faster and faster or slower and slower. Positive spike patterns were also found in patients with attacks of involuntary crying, laughing, or screaming and in patients with uncontrollable attacks of rage.

Unlike negative spike discharges, fourteen and six per second positive spikes are usually not temporally associated with the patient's clinical seizures. As a rule, during the clinical seizure, the electroencephalogram is normal and shows only low voltage activity such as occurs with attention. However, very rarely positive spiking is temporally associated with clinical manifestations, coughing in one case,[41] abnormal movements in another,[42] and a cold sensation followed by abnormal movements in another.[43]

If, as seems likely, fourteen and six per second positive spikes are evidence of disordered voltage production in a special part of the brain, and if one looks for the part of the brain that perceives pain and other types of sensation, that controls emotions, and that regulates visceral and vegetative functions, the thalamus and hypothalamus (diencephalon) are the only areas that "fill the bill." To some it may seem like a wild assumption to conclude that fourteen and six per second positive spiking originates in the thalamus or hypothalamus. However, similar reasoning led J. Hughlings Jackson to conclude correctly that a seizure with a sensory or motor march usually originates in the central area of the cerebral cortex.

The question may arise as to why diencephalic seizures are not temporally associated with seizure activity. One possible explanation is that such discharges, in a waking person, remain confined to deep structures. In sleep, thalamic centers drive the cortex, and one can see during sleep deep lying dysrhythmias reflected in cortical activity.

Positive spikes do not always have a precise frequency of fourteen or six cycles per second,[44] but as a rule they are close to these frequencies. They are usually bilateral but independent in the left and right hemispheres, and usually they show best in the temporo-occipital areas. They are characteristically a disorder of school age children and adolescents, and in these age groups they appear usually only during drowsiness or light sleep. However, among infants they occur in deep sleep, and among adults they often appear in the awake recording.

Fourteen and six per second positive spiking is a very common disorder, and it is often asymptomatic. It has been found in approximately 17 percent of unselected school children.[45,46] It tends to clear up spontaneously with increasing age, and it occurs in only 1 percent of random control subjects twenty-five to twenty-nine years of age (Table I). If associated with symptoms these usually decrease with increasing age. They disappear, normally, in late adolescence if not before. Positive spiking in general is a relatively benign, highly reversible disorder. Only a small percentage of those who have it are subject to convulsions or other seriously handicapping symptoms. Patients with positive spikes and symptoms based on such a disorder can usually be helped or entirely relieved of their symptoms by anticonvulsant medication.

The most common complaints of persons with positive spiking

TABLE I *

INCIDENCE OF CERTAIN ELECTROENCEPHALOGRAPHIC ABNORMALITIES AMONG 3,476 CONTROL SUBJECTS†

Age / Total Number of Cases	0-1 770 %	2-4 726 %	5-9 692 %	10-14 384 %	15-19 285 %	20-24 196 %	25-29 79 %	30-39 116 %	40-49 89 %	50-59 76 %	60+ 63 %
Hypsarhythmia	0	0	0	0	0	0	0	0	0	0	0
Petit mal variant	0	0	0	0	0	0	0	0	0	0	0
Petit mal discharges	0.1	0.1	0.1	0	0	0	0	0	0	0	0
Pseudo petit mal	0	0.3	0.1	0	0	0	0	0	0	0	0
Diffuse, nonspecific seizure activity	0	5.9	15.8	20.8	16.5	8.7	0	0.9	0	0	0
14 and 6/sec. positive spikes	0.4	0.1	0.9	1.5	2.8	2.0	1.3	1.7	0	0	0
6/sec. spike-and-wave	0	0	0	0	0.4	0	1.3	0.9	0	0	0
Psychomotor variant	0	0	0	0	0	0	0	0	0	0	0
Occipital spikes	0	0.8	0.4	0	0	0	0	0	0	0	0
Midtemporal spikes	0	0.3	0.8	0.5	0	0	0	0	0	0	0
Parietal spikes	0	0	0.1	0	0	0	0	0	0	0	0
Frontal spikes	0	0.1	0	0	0	0	0	0	0	0	0
Anterior temporal spikes	0	0	0	0	0	0	0	0	0	0	0
Small sharp spikes	0	0	0	0	0	1.0	1.3	6.0	7.9	6.5	4.8
Fronto-parietal spike-and-wave	0	0	0	0	0	0	0	0	0	0	0
Hemisphere spikes	0	0	0	0	0	0	0	0	0	0	0
Multiple spikes	0	0	0	0	0	0	0	0	0	0	0
Extreme spindles	0	0	0	0	0	0	0	0	0	0	0
S-3 diffuse	0.1	0	0	0	0	0	0	0	0	0	0
F-3	0	0	0	0	0	0	0	0	0	0	0
Minimal temporal slow	0	0	0	0	0	0	0	0	0	1.3	3.2
S-2 focus	0	0.1	0.1	0	0	0	0	0	0	0	0
S-3 focus	0	0	0	0	0	0	0	0	0	0	0
Runs of slow activity	0	0	0	0	0.4	0	0	0	0	0	0
Paroxysmal slow activity	0	0.1	0.1	0	0	0.5	0	0	0	0	0
Anterior bradyrhythmia	0	0	0	0	0	0	0	0	0	0	0
Mittens	0	0	0	0	0	1.0	2.5	2.6	3.4	2.6	0
Asymmetry	0	0.1	0.1	0	0	0	0	0	0	0	0
Asynchrony	0	0	0	0	0	0	0	0	0	0	0

* From Gibbs, F.A. and Gibbs, E.L.: Atlas of Electroencephalography. Vol. 3. Reading, Addison-Wesley Co., 1964.

† Persons without significant diseases, constituting a representative sample of the general "normal" population.

are headaches, dizziness, and attacks of nausea and vomiting. A small percentage of patients with fourteen and six per second positive spikes (or related patterns, see below) have one or more of the following: episodic pain in other parts of the body than the head, paresthesias, illusions, episodes of visceral and vegetative disorder, attacks of sweating, shivering, involuntary crying, laughing, or screaming, palpitation of the heart, respiratory distress, and emotional outbursts. Mentally retarded children commonly have fourteen and six per second positive spikes, but this pattern does not correlate with mental retardation;[47] it correlates with the episodic symptoms referred to above.

Fortunately, rage attacks are a rare expression of fourteen and six disorder, but occasionally they produce disastrous results. One patient had enough warning to isolate himself from everyone when he felt an attack coming on, but another, not so fortunate, shot his young son, and another (a child) shot his mother.[48,49] The diencephalon is a compact area, and diencephalic epilepsy can take many forms. Fourteen and six per second positive spiking does not pinpoint the site of origin or the direction of spread. A patient with this disorder may have several types of episode, but whatever type or types he has had in the past, he is likely to have them in the future. However, just as the first convulsion may be extremely violent, so a first epileptic rage attack may be murderous. A person with diencephalic epilepsy can have an attack of rage that is accurately directed and appears to be purposeful. His furor may be triggered by someone or something; it may last for several hours. It may or may not be followed by unconsciousness or sleep.

It would be a great injustice to epileptics in general to regard them as potential murderers, and the same statement holds for persons with fourteen and six per second positive spikes. This pattern is extremely rare among murderers, either juvenile or adult. Epilepsy is a statistically insignificant cause of murder, but the fact remains that it can be a cause.

Two other relatively rare patterns are associated with identical symptoms; these are six per second spike-and-wave discharges,[50,51] first described as "spike-and-wave phantom,"[52] and a rarer pattern, the psychomotor variant discharge.[53,54] Both patterns have strong six per second rhythms with a sharp positive component, and both are commonly found in combination with fourteen and six second positive spiking. Unlike fourteen and six per second positive spikes, these two related patterns are more common among adults than among children. They are illustrated in Figures 13 and 14.

The wave form of the six per second spike-and-wave resembles the three per second spike-and-wave of petit mal, particularly when it occurs in young children, for in the younger age group it is likely to be slower, approximately four per second, and of relatively high voltage. Another point of similarity is that, like the three per second spike-and-wave, it is more common among females than among males. (All other types of discharge are more common among males.) Still another resemblance is that in some cases it can be precipitated by hyperventilation and by photic stimulation. It usually is brief and bilaterally synchronous, but it can be unilateral. In adults the voltage is in general lower than in children.

In contrast, the psychomotor variant discharge usually shows best in the midtemporal area, and if bilateral, the discharges are independent in the left and right temporal lobes. It is present almost exclusively during drowsiness, and consists of runs of four to seven per second notched waves with a strong positive component, rather than the single negative spikes in the anterior temporal region characteristic of the interseizure recording of psychomotor epileptics.

These so-called diencephalic patterns have been the subject of much controversy. Some authorities insist that they have no clinical significance.[55-58] In general these abnormalities indicate only mild disorder, less severe than that associated with focal slowing or high voltage negative spiking. However, these patterns do correlate with states of ill health and with certain special types of symptomatology.[45] They are twice as common in medical-legal, post-traumatic cases as they are in a random sample of the general population, matched for age with the medical-legal, post-traumatic group.[59] They are twice as common in post-traumatic cases that are symptomatic as they are in post-

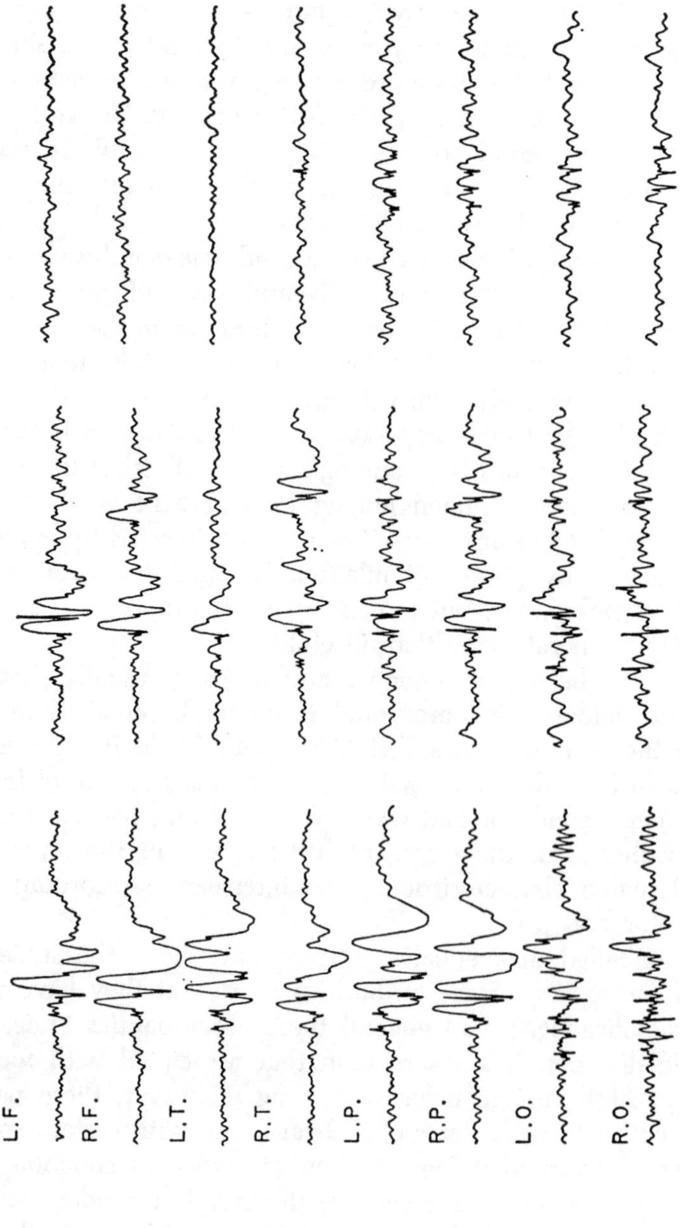

Figure 13. Six per second spike-and-wave discharge.

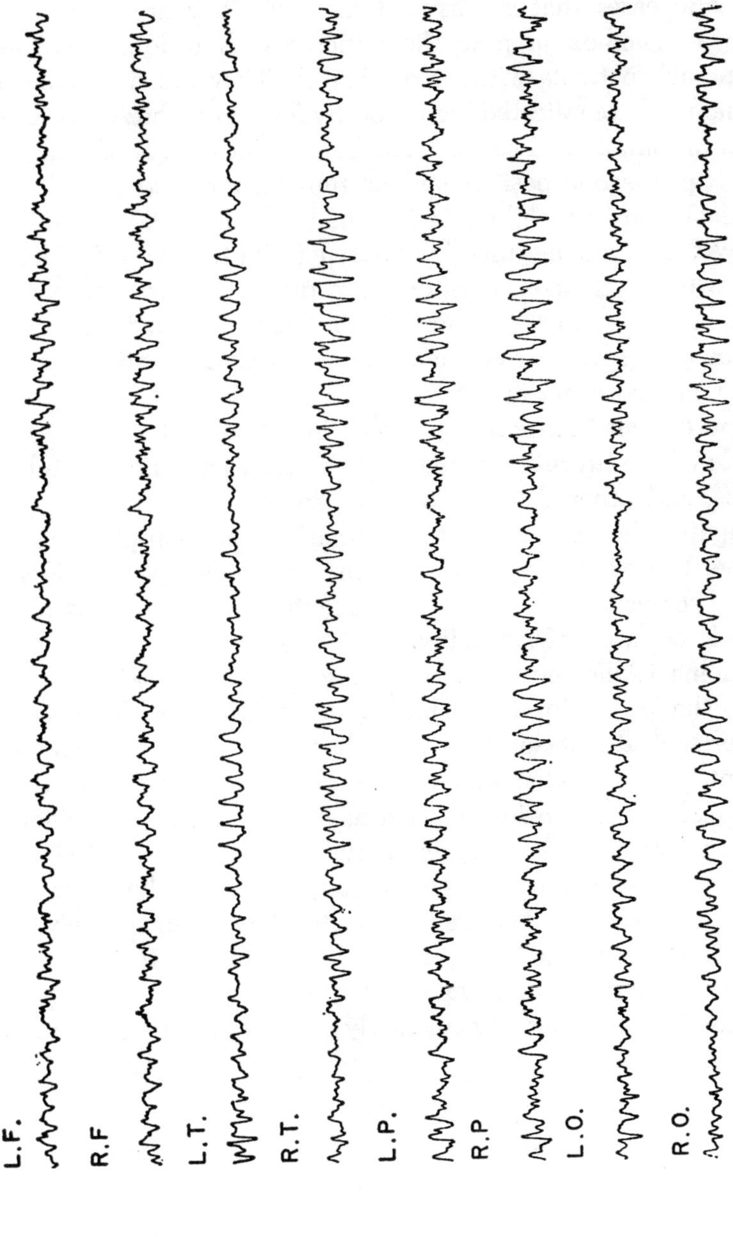

Figure 14. Psychomotor variant discharge.

traumatic cases that are asymptomatic.[10] They are more than twice as common in postpolio patients with residuals as they are in such patients without residuals.[10] They are five times as common in complicated cases of Sydenham's chorea as they are in uncomplicated cases.[10] The highest incidences of fourteen and six per second positive spiking thus far reported were found by Glenn[60] among children with duodenal ulcer (80%) and by Reilly *et al.*[61] among allergic children (60%). A high incidence of this dysrhythmia occurs in other disorders, for example, in muscular dystrophy[62,63] and Huntington's chorea.[10] For some unknown reason, fourteen and six per second positive spiking almost never occurs in mongoloids.[64]

How can an "abnormality" occur in 20 percent of a random sample of the juvenile population? In times past, rickets, tuberculosis, and other diseases occurred in at least as high a percentage of the general (not-so-normal) population. At present, in the United States, vascular disease would be considered normal for persons over forty if percentage incidence was made the sole criterion of normality.

Trauma is the most common cause of diencephalic types of dysrhythmia, i.e. fourteen and six per second positive spiking, six per second spike-and-wave discharges, and the psychomotor variant type of discharge. Twenty percent of patients with these abnormalities have a history of head trauma, a higher incidence than in any other type of epilepsy.[10] Encephalitis is the next most common cause. In the majority of cases, however, the cause is unknown. The genetic factor has approximately the same importance as in other types of epilepsy. It is not uncommon to find several members of a family affected.[65-67] Tumors and cerebral vascular disease rarely cause these abnormalities.

Chapter XI

FOCAL EPILEPSY, EXCLUSIVE OF ANTERIOR TEMPORAL LOBE SEIZURES

Electroencephalographic studies have shown that Jacksonian seizures, starting with a sensory or motor march, usually begin in the area implicated by the clinical signs and symptoms. In some cases, however, a series of spike discharges may start at a distance from the clinical focus and remain subclinical until they spread to a motor or sensory area. Doubtless, many seizures that appear to be both clincially and electroencephalographically generalized or diffuse originate from a focus in buried cortex or in subcortical structures too deep to be detected with scalp electrodes. In some cases, also, the discharge may spread so rapidly that the focal origin may be overlooked.

A detailed study of the clinical seizure and an accurate description of its onset may point to a previously unsuspected focus, but electroencephalographic studies both awake and during sleep commonly reveal foci that could not be discovered by clinical means alone. In many patients, particularly those with cerebral palsy or those who have outgrown an infantile, diffuse seizure disorder (for example, hypsarhythmia or petit mal variant), multiple foci are revealed by the electroencephalogram. In such cases the clinical seizures are usually of the grand mal type, and the focal origin of the seizures is not indicated by the character of the clinical seizure. On the other hand, surprising as it may seem, some cases with clinical seizures that are Jacksonian have normal electroencephalograms even during the clinical seizure. This is hard to explain, but the most reasonable explanation appears to be that the discharge may be too small to be detected or lies in buried cortex or in a subcortical area from which there is no spread to the outer convexity of the cerebral hemispheres. In such cases, negative findings are not positive evidence of normality, nor do they indicate the absence of a pathological process. Meningiomas not infrequently cause localized irritation with resulting focal seizures, unaccompanied by electroencephalographic abnormalities.

A recent unexplained onset of seizures in an adult, especially when they are focal, raises the possibility that a tumor, cerebrovascular lesion, or atrophic process is present. Although the incidence of brain tumor among persons primarily referred for seizures is less than 2 percent, the incidence of seizures among patients with supratentorial tumors has been reported to be 30 to 40 percent.[68] It is lower among patients with cerebrovascular lesions. If focal slowing or marked suppression of voltage production is present, the chance of an acute pathological process being the cause is greater than if the focus consists of pure spiking alone. A normal electroencephalogram in a person with focal seizures does not rule out the possibility of a structural lesion, but weighs the evidence against it.

Most clinicians complain that the electroencephalogram shows not too few foci but too many and too high a proportion that are subclinical. Such foci are important for an understanding of epilepsy, for though at first they may be subclinical, they may later manifest themselves clinically as focal seizures or episodic localized symptomatology that has an epileptic basis. An epileptic focus, even though subclinical, is clear, objective evidence of localized cortical disorder. In some children with a subclinical epileptic focus but without clinical evidence of the epileptic disorder, anticonvulsant medication may greatly improve the child's performance.[69] It is also true that when, with increasing age, the focus disappears, parents and teachers may report that "Johnny is a different boy."

Focal seizure discharges usually consist of isolated single or sometimes multiple spike discharges occasionally followed by one or more slow waves. Sometimes the foci are bilaterally symmetrical and synchronous. This is particularly true of parietal foci. Temporal lobe foci are almost always unilateral; when bilateral, they are almost always nonsynchronous and independent.

During a clinical seizure with a focal onset, the scalp record-ing generally shows spiky activity which increases in amplitude until it builds up into a run, remaining localized if the seizure remains clinically localized, but spreading to become general-ized if the attack is transformed into a generalized convulsive seizure. In some cases, the beginning seizure activity takes the form of an increase in fast activity; this is particularly true of seizures in the central areas, and sometimes the discharge may consist of localized activity of increasing amplitude in the fre-quency range of six to ten cycles per second. Following a focal seizure, one sees, not uncommonly, flattening and/or slowing in the region of origin. This focal depression of function following a seizure is probably the physiological basis of the transient, localized or lateralized, postseizure paralysis (Todd's paralysis) that occurs in some cases with focal seizures. Localized slowing after what appears to have been a diffuse generalized seizure raises the possibility that the region showing the slowing was the one in which seizure activity originated.

As previously stated, generalized seizure discharges are characteristic of the immature brain and focal abnormalities, particularly in the anterior temporal region, are more charac-teristic of adults. This is partly because certain types of injury are peculiar to different ages, but most especially because the vulnerability of the brain varies with age. Occipital foci are most common among preschool children, and midtemporal foci, among children of school age. In a high percentage of cases, both types of focus are subclinical, and in many cases, the seizure dis-charge clears up spontaneously without producing any clinical epileptic manifestations. However, a child with focal seizure ac-tivity is seizure-prone, and there is always the risk that clinical seizures will appear later. Occipital foci are especially common in premature children and in children with eye disorders. Chil-dren with occipital seizure activity commonly have visual disturb-ances and eye defects.[70] Types of seizure that are not particu-larly common but which are strongly suggestive of an occipital focus are episodes of nystagmus, of amblyopia, or of strabismus. Visual hallucinations also occur in a small percentage of cases with occipital foci.

A midtemporal spike focus is particularly likely to produce localized clinical seizures, and these are ordinarily limited to the face.[71] Attacks of speech disturbance are usually associated with a midtemporal focus, and fear, either as a warning of a convulsive seizure or as a submaximal seizure, also points to the midtemporal area as the site of the seizure discharge.[72]

Parietal (central) foci are commonly associated with focal clinical seizures, but such foci are usually accompanied by signs and symptoms of localized neurological defects and deficits; children with cerebral palsy, with and without epilepsy, often have focal spiking in the parietal area.[73] Paresthesia is an especially common aura among patients with a parietal focus.

A spike focus in the frontal region, although rare, is usually unassociated with any specific type of seizure; adversive attacks may occur with frontal foci, but spikes in this area are most frequently associated with generalized convulsions without any specific type of onset. As with foci in the parietal area, frontal foci are particularly common in children with cerebral palsy. In such cases, even though the discharge may be subclinical when first discovered, clinical seizures are likely to occur eventually if the seizure activity persists. Fortunately, even in the presence of a gross structural lesion, seizure activity tends to subside with increasing age.[74]

Fifty percent of children who previously had an occipital lobe focus become free of seizures, lose their focus, and develop entirely normal electroencephalograms by the age of nine.[74] By the age of fifteen the same happy state is attained by 70 percent of children who previously had a midtemporal lobe focus.[71] If the anterior temporal lobe is not involved, 90 percent of all children with midtemporal spike foci develop normal electroencephalograms and are seizure-free by the age of fifteen.[71] In cases where the epileptic disorder does not disappear, it tends to shift to that area which is most commonly the site of epileptic activity at the age which the patient as attained.[74] For example, occipital lobe foci, if they do not clear up, tend to become midtemporal, and midtemporal spikes become anterior temporal, or the disorder may move into the thalamus or hypothalamus with the resultant appearance of fourteen and six per second positive spikes. The favorable prognosis of children with certain types of spike focus has for some reason been rather generally overlooked.

Medical treatment of focal epilepsy is like that of all other types of epilepsy except petit mal (see Chapter VIII) and infantile spasms (Chapter V). If pharmacological treatment fails and if the seizures are so severely handicapping that they interfere with the child's education and social adjustment, surgical treatment should be considered. The child should be referred to a specialist or a group of specialists who have developed a high degree of competence in dealing with such cases.

Chapter XII

PSYCHOMOTOR EPILEPSY

Some older authorities classified trance-like attacks and confusional episodes, even when associated with complex, apparently purposeful movements, as petit mal seizures. J. Hughlings Jackson called them epileptic equivalents.[14] The term *psychomotor seizures* seems preferable since they are true seizures, and petit mal is now reserved for the type of seizure discussed in Chapter VIII. Psychomotor seizures are most commonly observed among adults. They are associated with varying degrees of amnesia. As a rule, patients with this type of seizure have, between their attacks and particularly during sleep, a spike focus in the anterior temporal area (Fig. 15).[75] Many authors make no distinction between midtemporal lobe epilepsy and anterior temporal lobe epilepsy; they lump both together under the heading, temporal lobe epilepsy. However, as previously stated, midtemporal lobe epilepsy is characteristically a disorder of children, and it is usually associated with convulsions; on the other hand, anterior temporal lobe epilepsy is characteristically a disorder of adults, and the seizures characteristically consist of episodes of disordered psychic function.

As long as the negative spike discharges or spike and slow wave discharges are confined to one or both anterior temporal lobes, spreading only to the ipsilateral midtemporal and frontal areas, no clinical manifestations occur. It must be emphasized that such subclinical discharges are most likely to appear in sleep. When, in the waking state, the discharge spreads widely to involve areas outside the temporal lobe, it commonly produces high voltage six per second rounded waves and flat-topped four per second waves in distant areas (Fig. 15) and a clinically evident psychomotor seizure develops. Following

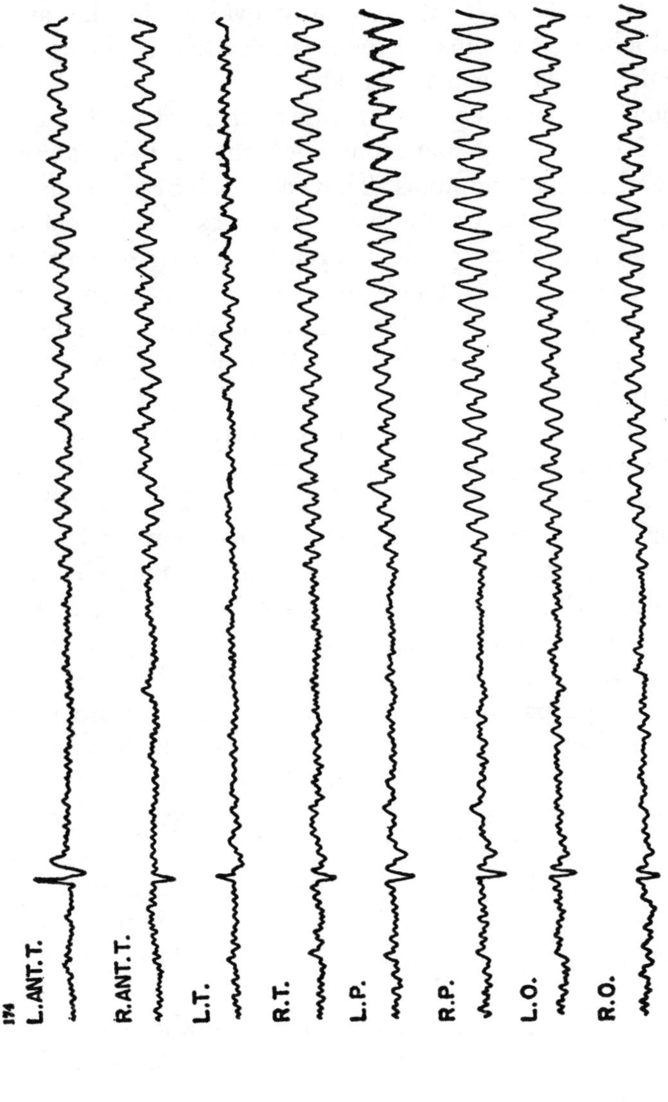

Figure 15. Anterior temporal spike focus (psychomotor type of focus), followed by a generalized clinical seizure discharge of the psychomotor type.

the seizure, focal slowing is usually evident in the anterior temporal lobe that originated the seizure; such focal slow waves may persist for days or even weeks.

Psychomotor seizures can manifest themselves in a great variety of ways. They may consist of one or more associated mental and motor symptoms. They can consist of a distortion of perception of self or of time; sometimes the patient has a feeling that a familiar place is strange (jamais vu) or that a strange place is familiar (déjà vu). Depersonalization or forced thinking may occur; usually the experience is unpleasant. Olfactory, visual, or other hallucinations may be present, but auditory hallucinations are extremely rare in epileptics. Seizures may be preceded by increased irritability, feelings of fear or rage, and by arrested or confused speech. An epigastric sensation is the most common aura. In the attack the patient may walk, run, sit, or lie down. He may do one or more of the following: stare, smack his lips, chew, swallow, mumble, rub his face, fumble with his hands or clothing, undress, act as though he were searching for something, run, dance, jump, sing, shout, cry, or fight. Actions tend to be repetitive and may appear to others to be purposeful, but speech and behavior are inappropriate. Autonomic manifestations may be present. In some cases, simple clonic or, more often, tonic movements occur, and the attack may terminate in a grand mal seizure. The patient is usually tired following the episode, and there is usually at least partial amnesia. Seizures vary considerably in frequency and length, and may remain undetected or barely noticed when they consist only of brief subjective feelings, staring, or isolated automatisms. They may be mistaken for dreamy states, somnambulism, intoxication, hypoglycemia, an abortive attack of insanity, hysteria, or simple amnesia. Distinguishing features are the frequency, relative briefness (in most cases), abrupt onset and sudden termination, the absence of an immediate cause, fragmentary memory, lack of complete awareness of the attack, and most importantly, a clearly abnormal electroencephalogram with an anterior temporal spike focus. A favorable response to a therapeutic test with antiepileptic medication is confirmatory.

Anterior temporal or psychomotor epilepsy is the most common type of focal epilepsy among adults; it is relatively rare among young children. Some cases are the end result of an epileptic process that started as an occipital focus in infancy, became a midtemporal lobe focus in childhood, and finally developed into an anterior temporal lobe focus in adult life. However, a high percentage of cases develop *de novo* in adults. As with other types of submaximal seizure, psychomotor attacks are often complicated by seizures of the grand mal type. In one study, 70 percent of patients with clinical seizures of the psychomotor type also had grand mal convulsions.[9] A few cases with an anterior temporal spike focus have only grand mal seizures. As prevoiusly stated, the combination of petit mal and psychomotor epilepsy is rare.

A high percentage of patients with an anterior temporal focus have more or less continuous personality defects or psychiatric disorder. Despite reports to the contrary, the great majority of patients with what has been called an "epileptic personality" are psychomotor epileptics;[9,10] patients with other types of epilepsy usually have normal personalities. Psychomotor epileptics are often reported to be "psychoneurotic," "obsessive-compulsive," "paranoid," "depressive," "psychotic," or "schizophrenic." Institutionalized patients bearing the diagnosis "epilepsy with psychosis" usually have psychomotor epilepsy and can be shown to have an anterior temporal lobe focus.[76] Often the psychiatric symptoms are more prominent and more handicapping than the psychomotor or grand mal seizures. Nonepisodic psychiatric disorder is an independent complication of the epileptic disorder; it is based on a different process, and it is sometimes intensified when seizures are controlled by medication. Cognitive and memory defects also are relatively common in patients with psychomotor epilepsy. As might be expected, when both anterior temporal lobes are involved, the seizures are usually more numerous and more severe than when the disorder is unilateral. Nonictal psychiatric disorder is also more common in the bilateral cases.

The etiology of anterior temporal lobe epilepsy is, like that of other epileptic disorders, nonspecific, and hereditary factors have about the same importance as in other types of epilepsy (Fig. 8). Trauma and encephalitis are the most common presumptive causes. A small percentage of cases are caused by cerebral vascular disease and by cerebral neoplastic disease. When a clearly defined slow wave focus or marked slowing is present in the anterior temporal area, especially during an awake recording, with or without spike discharges, and when a recent seizure has not occurred, the possibility of a structural lesion should be seriously considered. Certain authorities have suggested that in some cases the arteries at the base of the brain are pinched against the tentorium during a difficult birth and that this results in deficient blood supply to the temporal lobe and incisural sclerosis.[77] Difficult birth and birth complications undoubtedly produce epilepsy, but there is no evidence that they tend to produce psychomotor epilepsy. A history of difficult birth is less common in patients with anterior temporal lobe epilepsy than among patients with any other type of single area focus.[10] It is highest among persons with parietal lobe spiking and next highest among those with an occipital focus. Even patients with frontal spikes have a higher incidence of difficult birth than persons with anterior temporal spiking. Among patients with multiple foci of spike seizure activity, a history of difficult birth is highest of all, higher than in any other type of focal abnormality; it is more than five times higher than among patients with an anterior temporal spike focus.

Anterior temporal spikes usually persist for long periods and they do not tend to clear up with increasing age as do midtemporal spikes. When antiepileptic medications fail to produce benefit, surgery should be considered. If surgical removal of the focus is contemplated, the surgeon should have specialized competence in this type of operation. He will be guided by the electroencephalographic findings and will use repeated sleep recordings from the scalp before operation; possibly, he may also record from implanted electrodes in the depths of the brain and from the exposed brain at the time of operation. The more complete the removal of the epileptogenic cortex, the better the clinical results, but of course, there are practical limits.

Unfortunately, severe cases are usually bilateral, and radical bilateral temporal lobectomy, sufficient to remove all the discharging areas, is likely to produce severe defects of judgment and impairment of memory.[78-80] In bilateral cases, unilateral temporal lobecotmy gives good control of seizures in only one third of cases, but in selected cases it may still be indicated. When the focus is unilateral, surgery eliminates seizures in 50 to 70 percent of cases.[81-83] Because seizures can occur postoperatively and subside later, anticonvulsant therapy is usually continued for at least one year after surgery. Medication may eventually be reduced or withdrawn, provided clinical and electroencephalographic results are favorable.

Chapter XIII

SEIZURES PRECIPITATED BY SENSORY STIMULATION

Most epileptic seizures occur spontaneously without obvious, immediate, precipitating cause. In rare cases, however, a variety of factors precipitate or trigger the attack. In such cases the patient has a predisposition to seizures, and normally, he is subject to spontaneous seizures, as well as to triggered attacks. (For a discussion of seizures produced by systemic disturbances, see hypoglycemia, p. 72, hypocalcemia, p. 73, and uremia, p. 90.) The incidence of cases with triggered seizures has been reported to be 5 to 7 percent of all epileptics.[3] Precipitated seizures are sometimes referred to as *reflex epilepsy.*

The sensory modalities through which seizures may be induced are visual, auditory, somatic, and in some very rare and questionable instances, olfactory, gustatory, visceral, and vestibular. Genetic, biochemical, metabolic, and focal pathological processes can result in a lowering of the threshold for seizures in a specific area with the result that specific peripheral stimuli become epileptogenic. Such factors as the suddenness or unexpectedness of the stimulus are important; in others a rhythmic component is necessary, and in still others, complex psychic features are needed for the stimulus to be effective. The degree of concentration and the emotional setting, fatigue, and conditioning are all factors that can influence the susceptibility of patients to trigger seizures. Some patients report that they can inhibit their seizures by conditioning, by mental concentration, or by self-applied specific sensory stimulation. Deconditioning has been tried as a practical therapeutic method.[84]

Photically-induced seizures are the most common form of triggered epilepsy; they are especially common among children.

Attacks are usually precipitated by a sudden increase or decrease in light intensity, by a flickering light (commonly at a frequency of 10–15 cps), from visual patterns with contrasting light and dark areas, and from pictorial or reading material. Television, especially in countries where the scannnig rate and lines per inch are lower than in the United States, has been reported to induce epileptic seizures. In some cases the patient compulsively induces the seizure himself; this is especially common in susceptible retarded children, but it can occur in children of normal intelligence.

Petit mal and myoclonic seizures are the types most often reported as resulting from visual stimulation.

In the laboratory photic stimulation often produces abnormal response in the electroencephalogram; usually the electroencephalogram shows bursts of spikes and spike-and-wave discharges when such factors as light intensity, duration of stimulation, flicker frequency, and in some cases, color and attention are suitably adjusted.[38] However, sensitivity varies widely among epileptics, and "abnormal" responses can be obtained from a considerable proportion of healthy control subjects. Visually-precipitated seizures often respond poorly to anticonvulsant medication. In some cases dark glasses or tinted Polaroid lenses are effective in reducing seizures in patients with this type of epilepsy.

Audiogenic seizures are rarer than photogenic; they occur among susceptible epileptics with a sudden change of intensity of sound, with a startling or disturbing noise, and in some cases, with a sudden silence. In rare cases they are precipitated by intermittent auditory stimulation. Musicogenic seizures are extremely rare; the patient is usually an adult who is musically oriented. The seizures occur without startle and upon recognition of a particular type of music, instrumental or vocal. Seizures of auditory origin are most often akinetic or myoclonic, although psychomotor, petit mal, and even grand mal seizures have been reported. In these, as in other cases of seizures precipitated by sensory stimulation, the patient usually has spontaneous as well as induced seizures. Some patients without a clinical history of audiogenic seizures show subclinical electro-encephalographic abnormalities with auditory stimulation. Anticonvulsant medication is usually effective in audiogenic epilepsy. In some cases, reduced sensitivity results from continued exposure, from psychotherapy, or from deconditioning techniques.[84] In a few cases, focal lesions in the temporal lobe have been reported.

Somatosensory-induced seizures may be produced, or sometimes inhibited, by sudden tactile stimulation, such as a touch, tapping, rubbing, or pressure on a specific area of the head, extremities, or trunk. These effects can be obtained with merely the expectation of stimulation. A few authors have reported seizures precipitated by movement of an extremity, especially if sudden or if the subject is tense. Somatosensory seizures are often very frequent, with an onset in childhood. They are usually focal or Jacksonian in character; occasionally, akinetic, myoclonic, or grand mal seizures are reported. Writhing movements, usually after a period of immobility, followed by quick movements, known as "paroxysmal familial choreo-athetosis," are a rare type of seizure disorder that may be triggered by movement. It is somewhat similar to Sydenham's chorea, except that attacks are paroxysmal and may be controlled with Dilantin. Treatment of somatosensory attacks is usually difficult, but in cases with a localized lesion, surgical removal may lead to complete relief.

Some unusual, and in many instances unconfirmed, cases have been reported where seizures were precipitated by olfactory and gustatory stimulation (although such phenomena do occur as auras), by caloric stimulation of the semicircular canals, and by visceral stimulation (possibly related to cough syncope). Constipation has been considered a precipitating cause of seizures, especially by mothers who rely on control by enema, but many physicians believe that constipation does not precipitate seizures; it commonly results from the use of anticonvulsant drugs.

Chapter XIV

MASKED EPILEPSY, PARTIAL SEIZURES, AND AURAS

A wide variety of seizures fall under the heading *masked epilepsy*. Many types are comparatively rare, and others are surprisingly common, but all deserve special consideration because they pose interesting and often perplexing diagnostic problems for the clinician, especially when unassociated with typical seizures.[85,86] An electroencephalographic abnormality commonly found in adolescents with such seizures is fourteen and six per second positive spiking, as described in Chapter X. Also found in such cases, but more usually in adults, is six per second spike-and-wave activity and a rarer finding, namely, psychomotor variant discharges. (See pp. 45 to 47.) All are associated with similar symptoms, chiefly headaches and dizzy spells, but a great variety of somatic, sensory, and emotional disturbances also occur in patients with these types of dysrhythmia. Anterior temporal or pychomotor epilepsy may be mistaken for hysteria or attention-getting behavior, particularly if the seizure is complex and the behavior bizarre. (See Chapter XII.) Certain disorders that are nonepileptic, but that may be misdiagnosed as epilepsy, are considered in the next chapter.

Some epileptic conditions, which are ordinarily easily identified, may in certain instances present a diagnostic problem that can be solved by the finding of a clearly abnormal electroencephalogram. Among infants, one or more of the following may be expression of a seizure disorder associated with either hypsarhythmia or petit mal variant: recurrent, sudden, brief attacks of colic; stiffness with flexion of the head and body; unusual movements; excessive tremulousness and twitching; or spells of apnea and cyanosis. (See Chapters V and VII.) Unexplained, repetitive episodes of head nodding or falling in an infant or young child can be a result of epilepsy; in such cases the electroencephalographic abnormality that is usually found is petit mal variant. Not infrequently, thalamic or hypothalamic epilepsy, psychomotor seizures, or even true petit mal seizures may be mistaken for "simple dizzy spells," "fainting," "embarrassment," "hysteria," "behavior disorder," "inattentiveness," or "daydreaming." Very brief bursts of seizure activity, especially of the petit mal type, are sometimes associated with subtle alterations in behavior or performance. Prolonged attacks of psychomotor epilepsy or petit mal status with accompanying confusion may be misinterpreted as intoxication or a psychotic state.

Among some patients, especially those whose primary seizures are controlled by anticonvulsant medication, or those who are experiencing their first symptoms, a prolonged premonition of an attack or the immediate warning of an impending seizure may occur while the patient is still completely conscious. Such prodromal symptoms, or auras, may be the only symptom experienced, and they may be the only clue to the portion of the cerebrum presumed to be originally affected by the seizure discharges. Unless recognized for what they are, these symptoms may be misinterpreted by the physician if he has no other information on hand. Gastric auras are the most common. Often the sensation is described as "gas on the stomach," but the aura may be ill-defined, and some patients have sensations which they are unable to describe. Distorted perception or even hallucinations, visual, olfactory, sensory, and very rarely, auditory, can occur as warnings or as partial seizures. As stated in Chapter XII, psychic disturbances or illusions as a warning are most common among patients with psychomotor epilepsy.

Emotional states or outbursts, especially if sudden and inappropriate, acute feelings of loneliness, strangeness (jamais vu), or of unreal familiarity (déjà vu) are likely to be associated with a focus or spike seizure activity in the anterior temporal area. Attacks of rage or temper tantrums, a sudden change in the apparent size of objects (micropsia or macropsia), a change in loudness or brightness, attacks of laughing and crying are usually associated with fourteen and six per second positive spikes, six per second spike-and-wave discharges, or psychomotor variant discharges. Feelings of fear or anxiety are likely to be associated with a midtemporal lobe focus. Visual disturbances, either as a warning of the spells or as a partial spell, occur most often among patients with occipital spike foci. Episodic impairment of speech may be associated with a midtemporal spike focus. Epigastric disturbances most frequently precede psychomotor attacks. Impairment of body image or, more commonly, unexplained episodic pain, sometimes associated with other periodic autonomic dysfunction, such as nausea, vomiting, pallor, sweating, or respiratory distress, may be based on an epileptic process. The patterns most often associated with these symptoms are fourteen and six per second positive spikes, six per second spike-and-wave discharges, and psychomotor variant discharges. Tingling or numbness in one side of the face, a limb, or one side of the body occurred as an aura among 26 percent of patients with a parietal spike focus.[9]

All of these symptoms may occur only as a detached symptom, as an abortive seizure followed by loss of consciousness or sleepiness, or as an aura followed by a convulsive seizure. Sometimes the warning, even though blotted out by retrograde amnesia, may be sufficient to allow the patient to seek seclusion or safety.[3] In most of the doubtful cases, the diagnosis can be confirmed by an electroencephalogram recorded awake and asleep. A favorable response to antiepileptic medication supports the diagnosis.

A premonition or prodrome of a seizure may last for hours or even days before the actual seizure occurs. It may be only an alteration in mood, a period of dullness or vague, subjective, sensory or visceral and vegetative sensations, a feeling of malaise, or a premonition that something unpleasant is about to happen. Some types of epilepsy are rarely associated with a warning. These are petit mal, petit mal variant, and pure grand mal. (See Chapters IV, VII, and VIII.) In some cases, a shower of myoclonic jerks or of petit mal seizures precedes a generalized grand mal seizure, and of course, localized involuntary muscle movements commonly herald the onset of a Jacksonian march.

Chapter XV

NONEPILEPTIC CONDITIONS RESEMBLING EPILEPSY

Breath-holding Spells

Breath-holding spells of infants and young children might be considered a type of rage attack, but they are essentially benign and are not classified as epilepsy. They are due to cerebral hypoxia secondary to a spontaneous Weber-Valsalva maneuver. Frequency varies considerably; spells occur most commonly between the ages of six months and one year, and rarely after age six. They are precipitated by an acute emotional upset with anger, frustration, fear, injury, or pain. This is followed by intense crying; then the breath is held, and the child attempts to exhale against a closed glottis. When apnea persists beyond twenty or more seconds, cyanosis, rigidity, and sometimes opisthotonos with unconsciousness follow. There may be some brief clonic convulsive movements, but severe convulsions do not occur in these cases. Recovery usually takes only minutes, but may take hours following longer attacks.

The mechanism, which is circulatory, is as follows: when the child, after a series of deep breaths, attempts to exhale against a closed glottis, he raises his intrathoracic pressure and forces blood out of the great veins leading to the right heart. The heart cannot fill, and the blood pressure falls precipitously as the heart beats empty. With loss of consciousness the muscles relax, the heart fills, and the blood pressure rises again. The electroencephalogram during attacks produced in this manner shows no seizure discharges; it is usually normal at all times, except during the breath-holding spell itself, when transitory slow waves, occasionally followed by flattening, are present.[87] In contrast, children with epilepsy almost always have abnormal electroen-

66

cephalograms. There is no precipitating factor or intense crying; apnea and cyanosis do not precede, but occur late in the seizure.

The treatment of breath-holding spells is difficult. Some physicians prescribe maintenance doses of phenobarbital, while others believe that this is of little value. The long range prognosis is excellent; the condition is essentially benign. The main idea to remember is that, like so many ills, "this too will pass."

Orthostatic Syncope

Orthostatic syncope is not epilepsy, and it is not usually difficult to distinguish from epilepsy.[88] Confusion arises largely because "fainting spell" is a euphemism which the patient, the family, and sometimes the physician use to cover a socially unacceptable diagnosis.

In an ordinary faint, due to a critical fall in blood pressure, the patient usually has a warning of light-headedness, nausea, and a feeling of weakness in the knees. He wants to lie down and usually tries to do so. His face is pale, and there is usually a cold perspiration. As a rule, involuntary muscular movements are slight or absent. If the electroencephalogram is recorded during a syncopal attack, a series of high voltage slow waves is observed; these diminish in frequency as they decrease in amplitude until the tracing flattens. If extreme hypoxia persists for more than a few seconds, brief clonic movements occur. If prolonged beyond ten seconds, tonic spasm in extension is likely to develop. If the cerebral anemia is brief, the normal electrical activity of the cortex returns quickly.

In persons who faint easily a critical fall in blood pressure, such as occurs with postural hypotension, can often be demonstrated after prolonged quiet standing or with the aid of a tipping-table. In some instances, the sight of blood, fear, or grief triggers a cardiovascular reaction that results in syncope. Fainting at the sight of blood is so common that it seems possible that, like "freezing" in the rabbit, fainting has had survival value in the course of evolution. A drop in blood pressure and falling to the ground in a semblance of death may be life-saving under some circumstances, even if the spilled blood belonged to someone else.

"Fainting attacks" which occur while the patient is lying down are not likely to be true syncope; they are likely to be thalamic or hypothalamic epilepsy or psychomotor seizures (anterior temporal lobe epilepsy); these are the forms of epilepsy that are most often confused with orthostatic syncope. Headache and somnolence are rare after orthostatic syncope and common after epileptic seizures. Loss of consciousness with tongue biting and urinary or fecal incontinence are presumptive evidence of epilepsy and argue strongly against syncope.

Carotid Sinus Syncope

A hyperactive carotid sinus reflex is relatively common, but associated syncope is uncommon. It may closely resemble epilepsy, particularly in cases where a moderate amount of convulsive movement is associated with the syncope; however, severe tonic-clonic convulsions do not occur in this condition.[89]

There are three varieties of pathological carotid sinus reflex: (a) cardiac, associated with bradycardia or asystole; (b) vasomotor, associated with vasodilation and no asystole; and (c) the least common form, cerebral or central, unassociated with a significant change in heart rate or in blood pressure.[90] The last type may be a rare form of reflex epilepsy with the carotid sinus or other neighboring structures acting as a trigger.[91] The same patient may have more than one type. The lesion most often responsible is an atherosclerotic plaque in the neighborhood of the carotid body, often with associated narrowing of cranial and extracranial vessels.

In testing for a hyperactive carotid sinus reflex,[91] the patient should be seated, and the region of the carotid bifurcation should be briefly and gently massaged, first on one side and then on the other, never on both sides at once. If symptoms result from this procedure, it becomes important to make sure that they are not due merely to compression of the carotid artery. This can be checked by carrying out the same procedure over the carotid artery low in the neck. If pressure over one carotid sinus, but not elsewhere on the neck or on other parts of the carotid artery, causes dizziness, confusion, unconsciousness, or convulsive movements, a circulatory component is likely. The pulse should be taken, the electrocardiogram recorded, or the blood pressure recorded during pressure on the sensitive carotid sinus (preferably all three), and additional evidence can be obtained if the entire procedure is monitored with an electro-encephalogram.

In the interval between attacks the electroencephalogram is usually normal, but during the cardiac and vasodilator types of syncope, there may be a few slow waves followed by sudden flattening when the blood pressure falls to a critically low level. With the central type, even during syncope, there are usually no electrocardiographic or electroencephalographic abnormalities.[89-93]

Facial Tic and Involuntary Muscle Movements

Certain involuntary movements, such as facial tic, habit spasms, tremors, and clonic movements of reflex origin are not classified as epilepsy. They do not respond to antiepileptic medication and are unassociated with electroencephalographic abnormalities. They are doubtless produced by neuronal discharges, but these must be quantitatively or qualitatively different from those occurring in epilepsy. They remain confined to deep centers and lower levels and do not disturb cortical activity.

In some of these conditions, a satisfactory waking electroencephalogram cannot be obtained because of the constant muscle activity and movement. During sleep such movements usually cease, and sleep recordings are particularly useful for determining whether or not an epileptic component is present as a complication of a nonepileptic motor disorder.

Oculogyric Crises

Oculogyric crises are not associated with electroencephalographic abnormalities and are not classifiable as epileptic seizures.

Chorea and Athetosis

Choreiform and athetotic movements are usually too slow to be confused with the sudden jerks of myoclonic epilepsy. They are not temporally related to seizure activity, and they are not a form of epilepsy. The neuronal disorders on which they are based are not reduced by anticonvulsant medication, and they are usually unassociated with electroencephalographic abnormality.

Sydenham's chorea, a sequel of rheumatic fever, is a disorder of childhood. Usually in the acute phase of the illness, the electroencephalogram shows, in the awake recording, diffuse slowing predominately in the occipital areas. This persists in the postacute phase in some cases. Electroencephalographic abnormalities do not correlate with the presence or absence of choreic movements; however, in 65 percent of cases that are complicated by attacks of dizziness, headache, visceral and vegetative disturbances, or irritability and emotional instability fourteen and six per second positive spikes are found.[10]

Huntington's chorea, a hereditary degenerative disorder of adults, is characterized by irregular movements, speech disturbances, and dementia. A very low voltage waking electroencephalogram is common, and in some cases sleep patterns are abnormal. Forty percent of cases have fourteen and six per second positive spikes, the highest incidence of this abnormality thus far encountered among adults.[10]

Hemiballismus

Involuntary violent but brief jerking of one arm or leg, commonly referred to as hemiballismus, is unassociated with electroencephalographic abnormalities. The responsible lesion, as a rule, is in the contralateral subthalamic nucleus. Disorder in this deep structure does not disorganize or disturb the spontaneous electrical activity of the cortex. Patients with hemiballismus are not usually helped by anticonvulsants.

Spasmus Nutans

Spasmus nutans is nonepileptic; electroencephalographic recordings are normal. It occurs mainly in young children who have been kept in poorly lighted rooms. The head nodding is associated with nystagmus, but the head movements do not compensate for the eye movements; they are independent of each other. The disorder clears up in summer.

Familial Periodic Paralysis

In familial periodic paralysis, it is not the brain but the myoneural junction that is affected. The episodes of weakness occur because of recurrent critical diminutions in the level of blood potassium. This disorder is usually associated with a normal electroencephalogram and is not related to epilepsy.

Trigeminal Neuralgia

One might suppose that trigeminal neuralgia would be unassociated with either brain disorder or with electroencephalographic abnormality. This is usually so, but cerebral dysrhythmias are present in some cases, notably spike discharges in the temporal areas, homolateral to, but also contralateral to, the pain. This, together with the fact that in certain cases Dilantin prevents what appears to be typical attacks of trigeminal neuralgia, makes it seem likely that, in this condition, as in migraine, narcolepsy, gastrointestinal disorder, and neurosis, to mention only a few, an epileptic process can give rise to symptomatology that is usually on a nonepileptic basis.

Lightening Pains of Tabes

The lightening pains of tabes are a nonepileptic phenomenon.

Episodic Hypoglycemia

Episodic hypoglycemia may be caused by hyperinsulinism either with or without an islet-cell tumor of the pancreas. This disorder is often difficult to differentiate from epilepsy because, in predisposed persons with a low treshold for convulsions, hypoglycemia may precipitate epileptic seizures, especially of the petit mal type, but also of the grand mal or psychomotor types. Furthermore, congenital idiopathic hypoglycemia can cause hypsarhythmia in infants. The electroencephalogram in such cases is indistinguishable from that obtained in patients with these types of epilepsy when uncomplicated by disorders of blood-sugar regulation. Furthermore, repeated episodes of severe hypoglycemia can result in brain injury, with persistent slowing and sometimes spiking in the electroencephalogram, followed by recurrent epileptic seizures which are not temporally associated with hypoglycemia.[92]

The convulsions that occur during hypoglycemia are not preceded by or associated with the intense display of spike activity which commonly occurs in epilepsy. Bilaterally synchronous spike and slow wave complexes, usually maximal in the frontal region, but not as uniform as the classical three per second spike-and-wave of petit mal epilepsy, are often seen before hypoglycemic seizures.[93] These seizures occur most commonly at intermediate levels of blood sugar, which are not sufficiently low to produce coma.

The presence of a hypoglycemic factor should be suspected if the patient's attacks develop slowly, always occur several hours after meals, are preceded by hunger, sweating, or a prolonged feeling of lassitude, and if they are related to a history of diabetes or to insulin administration.

Seizures due to spontaneous episodes of hypoglycemia are rare. In order to make this diagnosis, appropriate studies of carbohydrate metabolism must be made, and a spontaneous decrease of the blood sugar level to 50 mg/100 ml or below must be detected immediately before or during a seizure. A presumptive diagnosis can be made if critically low values (below 50 mg/100 ml) are obtained repeatedly in the interseizure period. A lack of correlation between the degree of hypoglycemia and the occurrence of seizures may mean that factors apart from the hypoglycemia are primarily responsible for both the hypoglycemia and the seizures.[93]

Tetany

The spasms that occur with tetany due to hypocalcemia or to alkalosis are rarely confused with epilepsy because consciousness is not lost and electroencephalographic changes are usually minimal. When the disorder is severe, there is usually some associated carpopedal spasm; if less severe, the presence of Chovsteck's sign may point to excessive muscle irritability. Serum calcium levels below 3.5 mg mEq/liter are diagnostic. In some cases, slow waves may be present in the electroencephalogram or sometimes fast activity and possibly a few low voltage spikes, but muscle potentials often obscure these findings. The patient is hypersensitive to hyperventilation. In rare cases among infants, hypocalcemia is associated with hypsarhythmia (see Chapter V), and this may clear up when the calcium level is raised to normal.[94] Convulsions may also be present in older patients, but in uncomplicated cases of tetany, without a predisposition to epilepsy, seizures are by no means common.

Pheochromocytoma

Symptoms caused by pheochromocytoma can closely resemble those of diencephalic epilepsy, but in most cases, hypertension, which is characteristically associated with this type of tumor, gives a clue to the nature of the illness. If a screening test shows an abnormally high concentration of a metabolite of epinephrine and norepinephrine, 3-methoxy,-4-hydroxymandelic acid, in the patient's urine, this finding should be checked by chromatography. The electroencephalographic abnormalities are in general mild and nonspecific, and the electroencephalogram may even be normal in spite of severe clinical manifestations.[95]

Rum Fits

The convulsive seizures that occur after a severe bout of alcoholism are a withdrawal phenomenon, and not a sign of epilepsy.[96] During acute alcoholism, slowing of normal electroencephalographic frequencies occurs; this may persist for several hours even though the subject appears to have recovered. The interseizure recording of patients with "rum fits" is commonly normal, but may show nonspecific abnormalities, such as paroxysmal slowing, especially among patients with advanced alcoholism or psychiatric symptoms. There is usually no spiking to suggest that these patients have an epileptic tendency.[97]

If spike discharges are found in the interseizure electroencephalogram, if focal or psychomotor seizures are present, or if attacks have occurred which are not immediately related to drinking, the evidence would be against a diagnosis of "rum fits" and would favor epilepsy. Among persons who suffer from both epilepsy and alcoholism, the seizures usually begin at an earlier age than the alcoholism, but may be exacerbated by alcohol intake. In some cases, especially when the seizure is of the psychomotor type, it may be mistaken (as pointed out earlier) for drunkenness. Epilepsy sometimes results from severe head injury sustained during a period of alcoholic intoxication.

Convulsions After Sudden Barbiturate and Meprobamate Withdrawal

Patients who have been on high doses of either barbiturates or meprobamate (and possibly other minor tranquilizers) may develop a convulsive seizure when these are suddenly withdrawn. The dosage of such drugs should be reduced gradually over a period of at least a week. Withdrawal seizures are indistinguishable from the grand mal seizures of epilepsy; the electroencephalogram of persons with such withdrawal seizures commonly shows spike discharges like those seen in epilepsy.[98] When the person who has been on high doses of these drugs is an epileptic, sudden withdrawal may precipitate status epilepticus. A differential diagnosis between epilepsy and convulsions caused by withdrawal is difficult in addicts if they do not disclose their addiction.

Narcolepsy and Cataplexy

Narcolepsy is characterized by recurrent, often frequent, diurnal attacks of irresistible sleep. It is commonly associated with less frequent episodes of cataplexy, i.e. sudden, usually generalized weakness, commonly precipitated by surprise, and emotionally toned experiences, associated with laughter, crying, fright, or anger. Sleep paralysis, temporary loss of voluntary movement, often developing during the transition between arousal and sleep, or hypnagogic hallucinations at the onset of sleep may also occur with narcolepsy, but they are rare.

Narcolepsy and the associated symptoms mentioned above have been classified by some authors as forms of epilepsy, but this is misleading. In contrast to sleep-like epileptic seizures, narcoleptic sleep is characterized by light sleep from which the patient is easily aroused. He is usually mentally alert if the arousal is spontaneous or gentle, but may be somewhat dull and irritable if forcefully awakened.[3] Cataplexy, with its inciting emotional factors and full retention of consciousness, is usually easily distinguished from astatic or "drop" seizures which are associated with alteration of consciousness. The electroencephalogram in narcolepsy and associated disorders is usually normal between and during attacks. However, in our study,[10] patients under thirty years of age with narcolepsy had a significantly increased high incidence of fourteen and six per second positive spikes over controls of the same age, especially when the history was complicated by other episodic symptoms suggesting diencephalic epilepsy. The patients with "true" narcolepsy and normal electroencephalograms do not benefit from anticonvulsant medication. Their excessive somnolence commonly responds to treatment with amphetamines or Ritalin®,[99] and cataplectic attacks may also respond to such therapy. On the other hand, atypical narcoleptics, whose attacks of sleep are on an epileptic basis, have fourteen and six per second positive spikes, six per second spike-and-wave discharges, or discharges of the psychomotor variant type. They may not respond to these drugs, but may be benefited by Dilantin® and even by phenobarbital.

Nightmares and Sleepwalking

Emotional outbursts during sleep with loud, persistent crying, muttering, laughing, thrashing movements, struggling, or efforts to escape, as well as episodes of sleepwalking, are not usually epileptic seizures and are not ordinarily associated with electroencephalographic abnormalities awake or alseep. In some instances, however, they may be on an epileptic basis, especially if the patient is difficult to awaken. Anterior or midtemporal spikes and fourteen and six per second positive spikes, as well as other spike discharges, are more often present in cases with these symptoms than in normal control subjects, but when associated with definite seizure discharges, diurnal seizures are usually also present. If nocturnal sleep disorders are distressing to the patient or to his family, a therapeutic test with maintenance doses of anticonvulsants would be indicated even in the absence of demonstrable seizure activity.

Enuresis

Uncomplicated nocturnal enuresis in children has been reported by some authors to be associated with an increase in the incidence of electroencephalographic abnormalities. However, there is not a high correlation between nocturnal enuresis and either clinical epilepsy or seizure discharges, unless other complications, such as mental retardation, are present. Bed-wetting in childhood is rarely caused by cryptogenic epilepsy, and the same holds true for fecal incontinence. When loss of bowel or bladder control is on an epileptic basis, obvious convulsive manifestations are usually present.

Headache

In spite of statements to the contrary in the writings of such great authorities as J. Hughlings Jackson and William G. Lennox, migraine and epilepsy are completely different entities, genetically, etiologically, clinically, and therapeutically. As long as the diagnosis was purely symptomatic, there seemed to be a considerable overlap. However, with the advent of electroencephalography, cases of sensory epilepsy in which the seizure consisted of an attack of head pain could be differentiated from pure migraine. In the former, the electroencephalogram is usually abnormal, and in the latter, normal. Furthermore, with improved therapy, it became evident that certain drugs which are helpful in migraine are ineffective when headache is based on an epileptic process, and vice versa. Antiepileptic substances are without effect in cases of true migraine. Furthermore, headaches based on an epileptic process are likely to be associated with attacks of unconsciousness, convulsions, or other types of epileptic seizures. This, of course, is not true of migraine. Some patients with epilepsy have headaches as a postseizure phenomenon. These are not usually very severe and commonly respond satisfactorily to mild analgesics.

Usually a migraine attack builds up slowly with a long prodrome. Scotomas and fortification figures often initiate the attacks. The pain is commonly one-sided, and generally when nausea and vomiting are present, they occur late in the attack. In contrast, headache which is on an epileptic basis usually develops rapidly. There may be blurring of vision, but scotomas and fortification figures are rare; nausea and vomiting associated with an epileptic headache can occur at any time during the attack. Impairment of consciousness at the height of the attack raises a strong presumption that the pain is based on an epileptic process; so also pain, which involves not only the head but an arm or other parts of the body, raises a presumption that the condition is not migraine but epilepsy. In some cases of migraine, thought processes are slowed during the attack, and speech may become impaired. Regardless of these distinctions and differences, if what seems to be a case of pure migraine does not respond to antimigraine remedies, a therapeutic test with anticonvulsant drugs is indicated. So also, in a case with severe head pain which seems to be on an epileptic basis, if anticonvulsants are not helpful, antimigraine medication should be tried.

An adult with a history of typical migraine and a family history of migraine almost invariably has a normal electroencephalogram awake and asleep. He is more likely to have a normal electroencephalogram than an unselected control subject, and during a migraine attack the electroencephalogram is almost invariably normal. In rare cases, slowing is present during and following an attack; these are atypical cases of migraine. In such cases, if a significant amount of diffuse or focal slowing is present, or there is a marked asymmetry, with or without spikes, either during an attack or in the interval between attacks, the diagnosis of migraine is questionable. Children are less likely to have migraines than adults, and the occurrence of severe headaches in children creates some presumption of an epileptic or epileptiform disorder. When the headache is associated with dizziness, abdominal pain, nausea and vomiting, paresthesias, or emotional outbursts, the presumption is strengtened that the patient has diencephalic epilepsy and that fourteen and six per second positive spikes, six per second spike-and-wave discharges, or psychomotor variant discharges will be found in his electroencephalogram. The same holds true for adults who have headaches and one or more additional symptoms pointing to a thalamic or hypothalamic epileptic process.

Behavior Disorders and Psychiatric Symptoms

Head-banging, body-rocking, and similar rhythmic "habit patterns" in infants are alarming but essentially benign symptoms which are invariably outgrown; they are unrelated to epilepsy. Even in severe cases where one might suppose that the child's brain would be injured by the persistent head-pounding, the electroencephalogram is normal.[100]

Nonepisodic behavior disorders in children, for example, hyperactivity, autism, and juvenile schizophrenia, are in general unassociated with significant electroencephalographic findings. Of course, if the child is also mentally retarded, has cerebral palsy, or clinical epilepsy, this increases the likelihood that the electroencephalogram will be abnormal. The electroencephalogram can help to distinguish between those behavior disturbances which are and those which are not related to an epileptic process. The chances of finding an abnormality, such as fourteen and six per second positive spikes, six per second spike-and-wave discharges, or midtemporal spikes in children and adolescents are greater if symptoms such as episodic fear, weakness, headache, or speech disturbances are present. When outbursts of abnormal behavior, temper tantrums, or rage attacks occur in young persons who are ordinarily well-behaved and especially when they culminate in impaired consciousness or a convulsion, the disturbance is likely to be on an epileptic basis. The diagnosis is confirmed if specific types of seizure discharge which correlate with such behavior are found in the electroencephalogram and if antiepileptic medication prevents further outbursts. All this should not lead to the assumption that patients with severe forms of behavior disorder, associated with assaultiveness, eventuating in murder, have abnormal electroencephalograms. (See p. 44.) The great majority have normal electroencephalograms. Because fourteen and six per second positive spikes occur in approximately 20 percent of unselected control subjects of school age, their presence in a child murderer may be entirely fortuitous.

If neurotics with episodic symptoms or an "organic neurosis" are excluded, the incidence of electroencephalographic abnormalities among neurotics does not differ from that found in control subjects of the same age. Attacks of severe anxiety of the type that are seen in classical cases of anxiety neurosis are usually associated with a normal electroencephalogram both at the time of the attack and in the interval between attacks. However, episodic fear, anxiety, or tension states, particularly in children, can occur either as part of a seizure or as a seizure.

Psychopathy and sociopathy in adults have no significant correlation with electroencephalographic abnormality except in rare cases where epilepsy (particularly of the psychomotor or diencephalic type) is present. If psychomotor epileptics who become violent in their seizures are listed as *aggressive psychopaths*, diagnostic confusion is bound to result. Criminality is no more common among epileptics than among the general population. Criminal acts and murder are rarely committed in a seizure or in a postepileptic state.

The major psychoses are not related to epilepsy, and nonepisodic psychiatric disorder is not based on epileptic processes. Meduna, the father of convulsive shock therapy, thought schizophrenia and epilepsy were to some extent antithetic.[101] He theorized that convulsions might ameliorate schizophrenic symptomatology. There is certainly some truth in the theory, for convulsive shock treatment was found to be effective in schizophrenia, but more useful in depressions. When epilepsy is associated with psychosis, it is almost always psychomotor epilepsy. (See Chapter XII.) Sometimes the nonictal psychiatric symptoms in such cases are greatly intensified, if the epileptic seizures are controlled, and vice versa, and this is in accord with Meduna's theory that psychiatric and epileptic symptomatology are based on opposite types of disorder.

Paroxysmal Vertigo (Ménière's Syndrome)

Paroxysmal vertigo is characterized by sudden attacks of dizziness which may last a few minutes or several hours. Occasionally the attack is so severe that the patient falls to the ground. Most patients report that the entire environment spins around them, but some insist that they experience a sensation of intense dizziness without the feeling that things are spinning around them. Nausea, vomiting, sweating, and headache are common accompaniments of the attack. Tinnitus is often present between attacks, and patients with Ménière's syndrome usually have reduced hearing in one or both ears; in the majority of cases their deafness is of the nerve type. One might suppose that a search for a cause could be sharply focused on the vestibular apparatus and the eighth nerve. It is true that sectioning of the eighth nerve usually relieves the episodic vertigo, but tinnitus often persists. Such radical treatment is no longer necessary because modern otologists have developed a method whereby, with the aid of ultrasound, the vestibular apparatus is destroyed, but the cochlea is left intact.

The precise cause of Ménière's syndrome is not known. In spite of its paroxysmal character, it is not related to epilepsy. The electroencephalogram is normal during an attack. The best medical treatment is a low sodium diet. Perphenazine often helps reduce the dizziness. Sedatives and tranquilizers are sometimes useful, but anticonvulsants do not help.

The differential diagnosis between Ménière's syndrome and diencephalic epilepsy does not usually present serious problems even though dizziness, nausea, vomiting, and profuse sweating are symptoms of both. Electroencephalographers and epileptologists are rarely asked to aid in the diagnosis of Ménière's syndrome.

Hysteria and Malingering

The clinical history in cases of hysteria and of malingering, together with the electroencephalographic findings, usually makes it a simple matter to differentiate them from epilepsy. Hysterical seizures are rare at present, and the same holds for malingered seizures. The electroencephalogram between, during, and following hysterical or malingered seizures is normal. Spiking or other paroxysmal or focal abnormality is absent. Petit mal seizures are rarely mistaken for hysterical episodes because of their typical clinical features and the almost invariable presence of spike-and-wave discharges in the electroencephalogram during and between attacks. However, clinical psychomotor, diencephalic, and occasionally, grand mal or focal seizures are at times mistaken for hysterical or malingered seizures.

During an epileptic seizure in most instances, rhythmic slowing, spikes or spike-and-wave discharges are present, although in cases with a subcortical or diencephalic discharge, abnormality may not be evident in scalp recordings. Sometimes movement artifacts or muscle potentials may obscure the seizure discharge. One must remember that in the interseizure period seizure discharges are absent in 5 to 10 percent of epileptics, even with adequate sleep recordings. Normal interseizure electroencephalograms are least common among patients with petit mal and with psychomotor seizures; they are most common among adults with infrequent grand mal or focal seizures.

Nonparoxysmal abnormalities, such as slow or fast activity, correlate with a wide variety of symptoms, including seizures, but they cannot be considered confirmatory evidence of epilepsy in the absence of clearly identifiable seizure discharges. Howver, electroencephalographic abnormalities of any type are negative evidence of uncomplicated hysteria. Sometimes marked diffuse or focal slowing may be the only abnormality; such slowing is especially common after a seizure or in cases with frequent seizures. It may point to an acute or chronic pathological process; it may serve as a warning "red light" to anyone wishing to regard the case as purely "functional."

Serious difficulties arise in the differential diagnosis of hysteria and malingering from true epilepsy only in those cases where the patient is highly informed or has been expertly trained. The following two cases serve as illustrations:

1. A former trained nurse was brought from a distant city by ambulance after a week of what appeared to be status epilepticus. She had had bilateral burr holes made in her skull in the search for a subdural hematoma. Her electroencephalogram was normal during her seizures, after her seizures, and between her seizures. She slept normally, and all sleep patterns were normal. Her physician, convinced that this was a rare form of epilepsy, in desperation telephoned from a room adjoining the patient's to the research director of a large pharmaceutical company and asked what the lethal dose of a new intravenous anticonvulsant was. The patient, who had been convulsing continuously for several hours, suddenly ceased convulsing, propped herself on one elbow, and appeared to be listening attentively. Realizing that strong suggestion might be beneficial, the physician said to the pharmacologist, "Well, we have already used more than that, but we will have to use still more if her convulsions continue." The patient had no further seizures of any type. Subsequently, however, she developed a fever that ranged as high as 106 degrees, until an alert nurse found that she was holding the thermometer against a radiator.

2. A man, who had paid a "witch-doctor" to help him avoid the draft in the Second World War, had a seizure when he was arrested as a purse-snatcher. Draft examiners, suspicious of the genuineness of his seizures, had done a sensory examination with lighted cigarettes, but the patient had remained unresponsive. In the hospital his electroencephalogram was normal awake and asleep, even during seizures in which his pupils dilated and in which he urinated and foamed at the mouth. In these seizures the electroencephalogram showed only muscle potentials and

movement artifacts. After the seizure there was no slow activity, such as usually occurs with postseizure stupor. He could have succeeded in fooling his examiners if he had not been so proud of his ability and had not wanted it recognized. In the midst of a violent tonic-clonic seizure, while a doctor was examining his dilated pupils with an ophthalmoscope, he sucked in a great bubble of saliva and whispered in the doctor's ear, "How am I doing, Doc?"

Chapter XVI

CAUSES OF EPILEPSY

The causes of epilepsy are not peculiar or mysterious; they are the same as the causes of disorder in organs other than the brain. The things that can produce cardiac disorder also can cause the paroxysmal cerebral dysrhythmias of epilepsy, for example, trauma, infection, oxygen lack, tumors, abscesses, toxins, and metabolic diseases. However, the injuries that cause epilepsy cannot be too severe; they must produce intermediate, nonlethal degrees of injury. This degree of injury is not visible even with the aid of a microscope. It is molecular and does not show histologically.

Perhaps the word *injury,* as used here, will seem too strong; it may be thought of as necessarily connoting structural damage, but this is not so. *Harm* might seem a better word, but the difficulty arises not for want of a proper word, but because we do not usually recognize that an injury can result in serious chemical alterations in cerebral neurons without gross or even microscopically evident changes.

When neurons are killed, they do not produce epileptic seizures. Destructive lesions, the kind that show so clearly in gross pathological studies and in microscopic sections (for example, areas of softening, atrophy, and scarring), are not as likely to be associated with epileptic seizures as nondestructive lesions that occur when neurons are only slightly injured and irritated, i.e. when their intimate chemistry is upset, not enough to make them stop functioning, but just enough to make them function abnormally.

There are no characteristic structural changes in epilepsy; the pathology of epilepsy is not structural, but physiological. Epilepsy shows in the electroencephalogram but not in stained histological sections. This does not mean that epilepsy is not due

84

to *real* injuries. The injuries that produce epilepsy are less extreme but just as real as those that produce structural damage.

Around an area of destruction in which function has been abolished, there is commonly a zone of less severe injury in which seizure activity develops. So also during recovery a stage of intermediate recovery may develop which corresponds to mild injury, and in this state seizure activity is likely to occur.

To put this in a nutshell: epilepsy is what the brain does when it is slightly injured. For this reason, epilepsy is a common and also a treatable disorder. It is functional, reversible, and hopeful, in contradistinction to the classical neurological disorders, which are structural and, therefore, largely irreversible and hopeless.

Heredity

Without doubt there is a hereditary constitutional factor in epilepsy,[3,102,103] as there is in almost all other diseases. However, epilepsy can be produced by many types of injury to the brain, and what is inherited is, in general, not some form of epilepsy, but a greater or lesser degree of resistance to the types of injury that produce epilepsy. In many cases of epilepsy, multiple causes are operating; for example, a genetic defect in a given case may not be great enough by itself to result in "spontaneous" seizures; yet, when a minor head trauma is added, the congenitally vulnerable brain may develop an irritative, epileptic reaction to the injury.

The hereditary factor in epilepsy is of about the same magnitude as in diabetes; it is not nearly as great as in such diseases as hepatolenticular degeneration, phenylketonuria, or manic-depressive psychosis. By referring to Figure 8, it will be seen that, in general, one case of epilepsy in ten has a history of epilepsy among near relatives, i.e. siblings, parents, grandparents, aunts, or uncles. However, among patients with febrile convulsions, Chapter VI, one case in four has a near relative with a history of febrile convulsions. Fortunately, this, the most inheritable type of epilepsy, is also the most benign. (For a discussion of the possibility that epilepsy will occur in offspring, see p. 153.)

The percentages shown in Figure 8 are minimal. They were obtained by asking the standard question, "Is there anyone in the immediate family (brothers and sisters, mothers and fathers, grandmothers and grandfathers, aunts and uncles) who has had epilepsy?" Many people do not know much about their families. Furthermore, there is a strong tendency to hide mild cases of epilepsy even from the patient himself.

Clinical and electroencephalographic studies of identical twins[3,102] leave no doubt that hereditary factors increase the risk of epilepsy ten to fifty times. Even among persons with focal seizures[104] and among those with post-traumatic epilepsy,[105] genetic factors have been shown to be operating. Metrakos and Metrakos[40] have reported a 12 percent incidence of epilepsy in the near relatives of patients with petit mal and a 45 percent incidence of spike-and-wave patterns in the electroencephalograms of siblings of petit mal epileptics, when recordings were made between 4.5 and 16.5 years of age. A high incidence of diencephalic types of seizure discharge has been reported by several investigators among the near relatives of patients with such disorder.[65-67]

For many years a distinction was made between *idiopathic* and *symptomatic* epilepsy. Persons with the former were believed to have no brain injury but only a constitutional defect. With increase in our understanding, it has become evident that what had been called *idiopathic epilepsy* were cases in which no cause could be found. With improved techniques fewer and fewer cases are classifiable as *idiopathic*.

Is Epilepsy a Disease?

Some authors have preferred to speak of *convulsive disorders* rather than *epilepsy,* but these two terms are not synonymous. A large part of the symptomatology of epilepsy is nonconvulsive; convulsions occur only when the discharge starts in or spreads to a motor system. The majority of epileptics do not have convulsions.

Since there are many forms of epilepsy, perhaps it would be

better to refer to the *epilepsies* except when speaking of specific types. However, different types are often found in combination in the same case, and (as with diabetes and neoplastic disease) it is most convenient to include all forms, the pure types, transition forms, and mixed types, under a unitary general heading. Just as we do not say "the diabetes" we do not find it convenient to say "the epilepsies."

Some authors have concluded that because epilepsy does not have a specific etiology, it is not a disease but only a group of symptoms. The same objection can be raised to *diabetes, nephritis,* and *arthritis.* A special type of disordered function in an organ can be properly termed a disease.

Etiology

In the majority of cases, the cause of epilepsy lies in the past and cannot be remedied, but one of the most important tasks of the treating physician is to establish the etiology, if possible, and to determine whether or not the causal agent is still operating. If so, it might be eliminated or attenuated. When the primary cause is no longer operating, its identification at least raises the possibility of prevention in other cases. Only by making an etiologic diagnosis can public health measures be taken which prevent other cases and ultimately reduce the incidence of epilepsy.

Many cases of epilepsy begin in infancy or in early childhood and many of these have a history of difficult birth. In others, congenital defects or inherited metabolic errors are responsible. In still other cases, a toxemia of pregnancy or an infectious process complicated the pregnancy. German measles in the first trimester of pregnancy is a major cause of brain damage in the fetus. Only recently has it become apparent that such infection may produce little or no clinical manifestations in the mother and may pass unnoticed. It is now evident that subclinical infections in the mother can cause epilepsy, mental retardation, and neurological deficits in the child.

An epileptogenic injury may occur as a result of trauma or

hypoxia or possibly both during the birth process, and the injury may be aggravated by a delayed onset of breathing or by respiratory or circulatory insufficiency. It is often impossible to assess the etiological role of a specific perinatal injury, but there is no doubt that such injuries can, and often do, produce epilepsy. The role of Rh incompatability as a cause of seizures, mental retardation, and cerebral palsy is dealt with in Chapter XXIII.

Inherited metabolic defects, for example, phenylketonuria and galactosemia, as well as endocrine disorders, such as hypoglycemia and hypocalcemia, can cause seizures in young children. Such cases must be diligently sought for with suitable laboratory studies. Once found, there is a chance that they can be remedied before irreparable damage has occurred.[93-94] Rare, inheritable defects, such as the lipoidoses and tuberous sclerosis, are often associated with seizures. In the former, a ruby spot in the macula is a telltale sign, and in the latter, facial nevi (adenoma sebaceum), particularly across the bridge of the nose and on the cheeks, are diagnostic. In most cases, other members of the family are affected. However, as in all genetic disorders, occasional sporadic cases occur with no family history.

Porphyria

An inherited metabolic defect that results in the accumulation of abnormal hematoporphyrin in the blood and urine can manifest itself clinically by the sudden development of neurological or psychiatric symptoms. Pains in various parts of the body, confusion, psychotic behavior, and convulsions can result from an acute hematoporphyrin flare-up. The great danger is that the patient will be treated with barbiturates which intensify the hematoporphyrinuria; they are definitely contraindicated. Dilantin and Mesantoin® can be used with impunity. Sunlight and barbiturates can both act as precipitating factors. Portwine-colored urine is a diagnostic sign, but detailed biochemical studies on blood and on urine are needed to identify mild and atypical cases.

Pyridoxine Deficiency

Pyridoxine deficiency can produce epilepsy. Infants on a prepared food containing insufficient amounts of pyridine had recurrent seizures until the cause of their seizures was discovered.

Lead Encephalopathy

Lead encephalopathy is usually associated with marked electroencephalographic abnormalities, with seizures, and with mental deterioration and is often followed by death, unless the presence of lead is detected early by examination of the blood or excreta or by x-ray of the epiphysis. Plumbism is less common than formerly because of restrictions on the use of lead in paint and other items, but it still occurs. Children living in old, substandard housing all too often are victims of lead poisoning as a result of ingesting flakes of lead paint from walls, ceiling, or woodwork.

Subacute Leukodystrophy

Subacute leukodystrophy often begins insidiously; convulsive seizures are an early manifestation, and it is particularly likely to affect children. An electroencephalogram at the outset shows no specific abnormality, only slowing and spike seizure discharges, but in the late stages a characteristic, periodic discharge of identically patterned, high voltage slow waves develops.[106] This disease is invariably fatal, and the cause is not known.

Nephritis

Severe nephritis, with hypertensive encephalopathy or with coma, may be associated with electroencephalographic abnormalities, such as slowing, but negative spiking is uncommon, even in cases that develop seizures.[10] Toxemias of pregnancy and preeclampsia may eventuate in full-blown eclampsia with its attendant convulsive seizures, but these usually cease with the termination of the pregnancy. Slowing or, sometimes, increased fast activity may be present in the electroencephalogram in the late stages of a normal pregnancy.[107] The incidence of abnormality during and following parturition is much higher among patients with eclampsia than among those with preeclampsia or with a normal pregnancy. Sometimes such abnormalities are residuals of the eclampsia, but sometimes they preexisted and indicated a predisposition to seizures which became aggravated by the various complications of toxemia, hypertension, or metabolic disturbances. Subsequent seizures, usually grand mal or psychomotor, persist after parturition in only a very small percentage of patients who have experienced seizures during a toxemia of pregnancy. Among patients with a prior history of epilepsy, pregnancy tends to increase seizures in about one-half of the cases, but occasionally it decreases them.[3]

Allergy

Reilly *et al.*[61] have reported a high incidence of fourteen and six per second positive spikes and other diencephalic types of discharge among children with severe allergies. However, in general, allergic conditions are not closely associated with epilepsy or with significant electroencephalographic abnormalities. Episodic symptoms, such as headaches, dizzy spells, and syncopal episodes, occurring supposedly on an allergic basis, often turn out to be associated with spike discharges of some type, particularly fourteen and six per second positive spikes, six per second spike-and-wave discharges, or seizure discharges of the psychomotor variant type. Patients with supposedly "allergic epilepsy" generally have spike discharges indistinguishable from those seen in the majority of epileptics. Visceral and vegetative symptoms in epileptics are commonly presumed to be allergic when, as a matter of fact, they are manifestations of a diencephalic type of seizure discharge.

With severe anaphylactic reactions resulting in convulsions and coma, the electroencephalogram is extremely abnormal; the type and degree of abnormality (as a rule marked slowing) correlates with the clinical state of the patient at the time of the recording.

Pancreatic Tumors

An islet cell tumor of the pancreas can give rise to episodic hypoglycemia with resultant seizures indistinguishable from those seen in epilepsy and may ultimately produce epileptogenic damage to the brain, so that seizures may persist even after the islet cell tumor is removed. (See Chapter XV, p. 72.)

Miscellaneous

Other major causes of epilepsy, such as encephalitis, trauma, cerebral vascular disease, and brain tumor, are considered in subsequent chapters.

Chapter XVII

INFECTIOUS DISEASES

The importance of particular infectious diseases as causes of epilepsy varies with the geographic site, the prevalence of epidemics, the effectiveness of public health measures, and chance sampling. Radermecker has published an extensive study and review of clinical and electroencephalographic aspects of the encephalitides and encephalopathies.[108] The findings are different among infants, children, and adults and differ also with the type of encephalitis and with the severity of the disease, the extent of cerebral involvement, and the phase of the illness. Convulsions, generalized or often focal, may occur during the acute and post-acute stages and may persist or appear as secondary complications months or years after the illness. In general, cerebral sequelae of infection are the most frequent and serious in children and may result in neurological and mental deficits, seizures, or death. Next to perinatal injury, infectious diseases are the most common cause of seizures starting in childhood.

Primary and secondary disorders resulting from invasion of the brain by various pathogenic agents can be brought into sharp focus by the use of electroencephalography; this technique makes visible abnormalities that correlate with, but which are often not evidenced by clinical manifestations. Even in supposedly uncomplicated cases of infectious diseases of childhood the electroencephalogram commonly shows that the brain has been involved.[109] The most usual change is slowing in the awake recording with a normal sleep recording. The slow waking activity commonly disappears within one or two weeks after the onset of symptoms and is more or less independent of the degree of fever. Among the common childhood diseases, measles is the worst offender; approximately 30 percent of supposedly uncomplicated cases have diffuse very slow activity in the electroencephalogram during the acute and postacute phase of the illness.[109] If the electroencephalogram remains normal, the prognosis is excellent for recovery without central nervous system residuals. If it is slow during the acute phase, the prognosis is not so favorable. Complications, including behavior disorders and intellectual defects, may occur. Slowing persists for a year or more in one percent of cases. With the passage of time the diffuse slowing (if it does not clear up) changes to focal slowing or spiking or both. Many months, or even years, after a spike focus has developed the child may have his first convulsion, and unless the spiking clears up after that he is likely to have recurrent seizures.

In viral encephalitis, especially among children, extreme slowing, maximal in the awake recording, is common in the acute phase; subsequent development of spike seizure activity is not unusual.[10] If consciousness is impaired, slow activity is almost invariably present, but extreme slowing can be present in an apparently alert child. In very severe cases of encephalitis, periods of generalized flattening develop. Recovery is associated with an increase in activity and gradual return to normal frequencies, usually within a few days or weeks after the acute symptoms have subsided. Among children, slowing usually persists longest in the occipital region.

Spikes are uncommon during the acute phase of encephalitis, but clinical convulsions are common. Not all children who have convulsions in the acute phase continue to have convulsions and become epileptics afterward. Among those with convulsions in the acute phase, 41 percent subsequently develop negative spikes in their electroencephalograms, and at least half of these go on to have recurrent seizures. Although encephalitis can cause almost any type of seizure activity, including hypsarhythmia and petit mal variant, it rarely causes true petit mal. Single and multiple foci of spike seizure activity are the most usual findings in cases of postencephalitic epilepsy. Approximately half of patients who develop fourteen and six per second positive spikes as a result of encephalitis are asymptomatic, i.e. the dysrhythmia is subclinical. The other half have one or more of the various symptoms that are associated with fourteen and six per second positive spikes (Chapter X). Positive spikes are more likely to appear after poliomyelitis and Sydenham's chorea, if the case is one with unusual complicating symptoms.[10]

It is not always possible to differentiate between a simple febrile convulsion (see Chapter VI) and a convulsion incidental to the acute phase of a mild encephalitis. A normal electroencephalogram in the acute phase of a febrile illness argues against encephalitis. On the other hand, an abnormal electroencephalogram several days after a convulsion that occurred during a febrile illness argues against a diagnosis of uncomplicated febrile convulsion. If the recording is abnormal in the postacute phase of the illness, the prognosis varies with the type and degree of abnormality and its subsequent course, i.e. whether it disappears, decreases, persists or increases.

Rarely does immunization against childhood diseases cause severe allergic reactions and recurrent seizures. However, convulsions are more likely to follow an infection than an inoculation. As a rule, even patients with known neurological deficits, with seizures, and with electroencephalographic abnormalities show little adverse effect from various types of immunization.

Certain chronic forms of encephalitis are associated with severe electroencephalographic changes and seizures; for example, chronic subacute leukoencephalitis is associated with slowing and spiking and in the late stages with myoclonus and distinctive repetitive bursts of diffuse high voltage slow waves with some spikes.[106] Seizures are common in cases of Schilder's encephalomyelitis, and the electroencephalogram is usually exceedingly abnormal.[10]

If the meninges alone are involved by an infectious process, seizures are not likely to occur. In general, meningitic infections are not as severe as encephalitis, and the electroencephalogram is little, if at all, altered. However, the consequences of meningoencephalitis can be the same or worse than the consequences of encephalitis. The outcome in cases of meningococcal and tuberculous meningitis depends on the age of the patient and the effectiveness of treatment. Prognostically electroencephalographic changes usually parallel or precede clinical changes. In the post-acute phase, serial recordings make it possible to predict with some reliability the development of seizures from the continuing presence of spike discharges, and an imminent relapse can be predicted from the reappearance of slow activity.

A brain abscess is usually associated with marked focal slowing, but a distinction between a sharply localized infectious process (preabscess) and an abscess cannot be made electroencephalographically. Recurring seizures are a common consequence of both.

In central nervous system syphilis the incidence of convulsions and the amount of electroencephalographic abnormality varies with the severity and form of the disease; both are more common in meningovascular syphilis than in general paresis.[110]

The incidence of epilepsy as a result of invasion of the cerebrum by various parasitic organisms varies widely with the type of organism. Seizures are a rare complication of malaria; schistosomiasis may cause convulsions, as may also cysticercosis.[23] Cerebral involvement is unusual with trichinosis. Seizures may occur with histoplasmosis and toxoplasmosis. In general the electroencephalogram accords with the clinical symptomatology; the maximal abnormality is usually found in the vicinity of the lesion.

Chapter XVIII

BRAIN TRAUMA

The majority of persons with brain trauma do not develop post-traumatic seizures. This holds true even for cases with severe cerebral contusion and neurological signs of brain damage, and with diffuse or even focal changes in the electroencephalogram during the acute phase. However, the incidence of seizures following open or closed craniocerebral injuries is considerable and appears to be increasing, apparently along with the increase in traffic accidents and also brain wounds of war. The frequency of head injury varies with age, sex, and occupation. The frequency of post-traumatic epilepsy varies with the nature and extent of the injury, with the treatment, and with the patient's inherited seizure threshold. According to Penfield and Humphreys,[111] the incidence of epilepsy is the highest in cases of depressed fracture, meningocerebral laceration, and drained and healed abscess. Jennett and Lewin[112] reported that less than 10 percent of cases develop epilepsy after blunt head injury. Early seizures predisposed to late epilepsy in 25 percent of their cases, and intracranial hematoma carried a similar risk. A combination of depressed fracture and post-traumatic amnesia created an increased risk of persistent seizures.

In post-traumatic cases the electroencephalogram, when added to other data, is a valuable aid for diagnosis and prognosis, and it can also provide important medicolegal evidence. Serial recordings permit an estimate of the degree of injury and the rate of recovery, or they may reveal the beginning of an irritative reaction to injury which carries the threat of epilepsy. If recordings are made soon after the injury, subsequent studies may show a sequence of changes that point to a traumatic origin of seizures that may not develop until long after the accident. In some cases an accident is caused by a seizure, rather than the seizure being caused by the accident. If recordings made soon after the accident show no slowing, but only spiking, and if there is no change with time after the accident, this creates some presumption of the former. As a rule, the slowing that occurs immediately after the accident gradually diminishes, and the electroencephalogram either normalizes (in uncomplicated cases within 3 months), or focal slowing or spikes develop.[113]

Electroencephalographic findings vary to some degree, although not precisely, with the nature and severity of the head injury, with the interval since the accident, and with the age of the patient. During the acute phase, persistent severe focal slowing or asymmetry, in addition to diffuse abnormality, may indicate a circumscribed lesion and facilitate the early diagnosis of intracranial hemorrhage, subdural hematoma, abscess, or other complications. With severe injury some generalized slowing or flattening is usually present during the first several days; the changes are somewhat proportional to the degree of impairment of consciousness unless damage has occurred in the depths of the brain. Electroencephalographic abnormality tends to persist longer than the clinical symptoms, except when neurological symptoms are due to a destructive lesion. After three months or more the electroencephalogram may continue to show some residual slowing or depression of voltage production, or it may normalize. Persistent electroencephalographic and clinical abnormalities offer a poor prognosis; a normal electroencephalogram and persistent neurological symptoms suggest a bad prognosis as symptoms are presumably due to the destruction rather than the malfunction of cerebral neurons. Electroencephalographic abnormality alone, months or years later, indicates that some degree of impairment is still present that may result in late complications. Normalization of both clinical and electroencephalographic findings makes the prognosis excellent. Post-traumatic psychiatric symptoms and intellectual defects do not correlate well with electroencephalographic abnormality, unless seizures are also present.

Occasionally spiking, usually associated with seizures but not always, is present shortly following the trauma. Subsequent improvement and normalization often occur and suggest a favorable prognosis, but a similar abnormality may reappear even more than a year later, and repeated sleep recordings at long intervals are necessary to evaluate properly the prognosis. Seizures may be triggered later by an intervening trauma or infectious disease or by physiologic factors. Spike discharges, with or without focal slowing, fast activity, or reduced voltage production, persisting or increasing after a head injury, make the prognosis unfavorable; persons with these findings are seizure-prone. Jennett and Lewin report[112] that in 50 percent of cases with seizures following blunt head injury the onset is within the first year, but in some cases the seizures do not start until several years after the accident.

The location and type of electroencephalographic abnormality are influenced by the primary site of the traumatic lesion, but distant effects often occur in the depths of the brain or in a contrecoup position. Abnormality may also develop around scar tissue or on the rim of a bone defect or a trephine opening. Electroencephalographic findings after trauma are related to the age of the patient at the time of the recording. (See pp. 8, 9.) Seizures of all types may occur, including paroxysmal attacks that are at first difficult to diagnose. Minor attacks of paresthesias, pain, dizzy spells, blackouts, or localized twitching may progress to a generalized seizure, but genuine petit mal attacks are rare.

In general the prognosis in post-traumatic epilepsy is favorable. Major seizures following head trauma are usually infrequent among adults, but are likely to be more frequent and more severe among children. Masquin and Courjon report[114] that 65 percent of patients, especially adults without a history of alcoholism, recover from post-traumatic seizures in one to five years when receiving regular anticonvulsant medication. According to Walker,[105] favorable prognostic factors among 244 adults with craniocerebral injuries of World War II were early cessation of attacks, low frequency of attacks, and severe neurological deficit, regardless of treatment with anticonvulsants.

Because even one or two clinical seizures can produce irreparable social and economic consequences, prophylactic anti-convulsant medication may be indicated to prevent the appearance of overt seizures among post-traumatic patients who have not had a seizure, but who have developed spike discharges. Most patients with post-traumatic epilepsy respond well to anticonvulsant treatment; this should be continued until the patient is seizure-free and has had a normal electroencephalogram awake and asleep for at least one year.

Chapter XIX

CEREBRAL VASCULAR DISEASE

A circulatory breakdown causing either transient or permanent damage to the brain can occur at any age, but the young and the old are especially susceptible. Seizures are a common early and late symptom of cerebrovascular disease.

The electroencephalogram, when used in conjunction with other methods, can be a valuable diagnostic and prognostic tool for the confirmation and localization of disorder due to cerebral vascular pathology and for the detection of irritative reactions to injury which may result in seizures. The type and amount of abnormality present in the electroencephalogram are closely related to the stage of development, severity, extent, location, and degree of cortical involvement.

Subdural hematoma of the newborn causes convulsions in about 5 percent of cases. Similar electroencephalographic findings occur among children and adults with subdural hematoma, except that spike discharges and seizures are more common among children. The most frequently encountered and reliable lateralizing sign among patients with a subdural hematoma is a reduction of amplitude (suppression of voltage production), with or without slowing, awake or asleep. In cases with bilateral fluid accumulation, asymmetry may be present even when there is no marked difference in the size of the hematomas on the two sides. A normal electroencephalogram does not exclude a subdural hematoma, and a marked asymmetry is not specific for this condition.[115] Spiking, if present, is not a reliable localizing or lateralizing sign, but in postoperative recordings it provides prognostic information as to the presence of continuing abnormality and the likelihood of recurring seizures. Usually suppression of voltage production and slowing clear up within a week or two, after the subdural hematoma has been removed, but both may persist. A normal postoperative electroencephalogram awake and asleep suggests an excellent prognosis, particularly as far as seizures are concerned.

Vascular anomalies of the brain, hemangiomas, and congenital arteriovenous aneurysms can be epileptogenic. Recurrent seizures are common among patients with Sturge Weber syndrome, i.e. a hemangioma in the distribution of the upper division of the trigeminal nerve; in such cases there is usually an intracranial angioma which includes the meninges. Congenital arterial aneurysms of the cerebral vessels can cause seizures; after leaking they are particularly likely to do so. If the patient survives a rupture, damaged and dysfunctioning but still viable neurons commonly develop an irritative reaction to injury which eventuates in epileptic seizures.

A minor cerebrovascular accident or a sudden vascular insufficiency can cause sudden loss of consciousness without persistent motor or sensory defects and in some cases may be difficult to distinguish from an epileptic seizure. Such episodes are especially likely to occur among older persons. Diffuse or focal slowing or an amplitude asymmetry in the electroencephalogram raises a presumption of localized damage. Abnormality which decreases over a period of days or weeks strongly favors the assumption that the disorder was secondary to a cerebral vascular accident. In some instances, spike discharges develop and persist, and ultimately the underlying disorder may express itself in clinical seizures.

Usually a cerebrovascular accident has such a sudden onset that it can be easily differentiated from a tumor. In some cases, however, it is not easy to distinguish between a slowly developing vascular lesion and a tumor except by arteriography or possibly by ventriculography. A cerebrovascular lesion usually produces a more limited slow wave focus than a tumor, and if slow activity is present on the unaffected side, it often clears up in a few days. Usually a trend toward regression of the focus and general improvement of the patient's clinical condition is evident within ten days. Spikes and seizures are somewhat less common among patients with cerebrovascular disease than among those with cortical tumors. Old age, of course, is a time when cerebrovascular disease becomes a probable diagnosis, and the probability is increased if the patient has diabetes or hypertension.

Patients with chronic mild cardiovascular disturbances, moderate arterial hypertension, and arteriosclerosis usually have normal electroencephalograms or slightly abnormal ones with slowing or fast activity, usually minimal and diffuse but occasionally focal, especially in the temporal or frontal areas. In cases of epilepsy resulting from cerebrovascular insufficiency, small sharp spikes are common, and other types of spike seizure discharge are relatively rare. Small sharp spikes are frequently asymptomatic, but they indicate a low seizure threshold; persons with this abnormality are seizure-prone. (See Table I.)

Chapter XX

BRAIN TUMOR

Brain tumors are an important, but fortunately uncommon cause of epilepsy in adults; they are an exceedingly rare cause of epilepsy in children because brain tumors in children are usually subtentorial. All patients with seizures, particularly focal seizures of undetermined etiology, and with neurological deficits deserve careful study, but the notion that strenuous efforts must be made to detect a brain tumor as early as possible is incorrect. In the absence of signs of pressure and particularly in the absence of choked disc, expectant treatment is permissible. If a patient has no symptoms except seizures and no papilledema, an increase in electroencephalographic abnormality will warn of a possible brain tumor in plenty of time for definitive studies to be carried out. The routine use of arteriograms and pneumoencephalograms in all cases of epilepsy is unwarranted.

A brain tumor was found in only 4 percent of adults with epilepsy studied by Lennox[3] and in only 1 percent of 11,612 epileptics of all ages studied by Gibbs and Gibbs.[9] There were no cases of brain tumor among the 742 epileptic children studied by Bridge.[1]

Brain tumors are not as epileptogenic as is commonly supposed. Analysis of over one thousand cases of brain tumor, from the services of Harvey Cushing and Walter Dandy,[116] showed that even when the tumor is located in the most favorable area, i.e. the parietal or temporal lobes, it produces convulsive seizures in no more than 30 to 35 percent of cases. Penfield and Erickson[117] cite six authors who reported a 29 to 39 percent incidence of seizures in cases with proven brain tumor. When subtentorial tumors were excluded from the series that they collected at the Montreal Neurological Institute, 45 percent of the patients had seizures. This last figure is probably excessive because the reputation of the Institute as a center for the treatment of epilepsy doubtless attracted a disproportionate number of patients with brain tumor and seizures, while those with brain tumor and no seizures probably gravitated elsewhere.

Penfield and Erickson[117] and also Guvener and his colleagues[118] found that in general the slower the rate of growth of the tumor and the less its malignancy, the greater the likelihood of seizures; oligodendrogliomas rank highest in epileptogenicity, and glioblastomas, lowest. Meningiomas commonly show the least electroencephalographic changes. Acute lesions tend to show the greatest focal slowing, and chronic lesions, the most seizure activity. Seizure discharges alone, without focal slowing, are usually not associated with an expanding lesion. A gradual increase in focal slowing in serial recordings suggests an expanding lesion. A progressive decrease in slowing is strong negative evidence against a tumor. In spite of the fact that occasionally a patient with a brain tumor has a normal electroencephalogram, this finding in a patient with seizures usually means "no tumor."[10]

Increasing postoperative abnormality and, particularly, the development or persistence of spike discharges raise the possibility of clinical seizures. If a tumor causes recurrent seizures, they do not necessarily cease after the removal of the tumor. In some cases with a brain tumor and no seizures, the operative trauma creates conditions which, after a varying length of time, result in recurring seizures.

Chapter XXI

STUPOR AND COMA

Although the clinical signs and symptoms may be sufficient to distinguish stupor or coma that is and that is not related to epilepsy, the electroencephalogram is particularly useful for this purpose. If, in an unresponsive patient, normal sleep activity with biparietal humps, spindles, and slow waves are present, the chances are that one is dealing with postseizure stupor. Spike discharges, sometimes with focal slowing or with spike-and-wave patterns, gradually reappearing during sleep or following arousal, point clearly to the diagnosis of epilepsy and are strong evidence against stupor or coma of a more serious nature.

In some instances, *epilepsia partialis continua*, without overt but sometimes with perceptible convulsive manifestations, may be associated with marked electroencephalographic abnormalities and seizure discharges, and may masquerade as stupor or coma. Petit mal status can manifest itself as stupor, but usually fluctuations of consciousness can be detected, which point to an epileptic rather than a nonepileptic disorder. Similarly, psychomotor status may appear as a persistent clouding of consciousness, but the characteristic anterior temporal lobe spiking is diagnostic. Very prolonged periods (24 hours or more) of flaccid unconsciousness occur as a rare form of seizure in patients with fourteen and six per second positive spikes.

Chapter XXII

MENTAL RETARDATION

Mental deficiency is less frequently reported at present than in the past among patients with epilepsy, but the percentage of retardates in any large population of epileptics, especially if it includes children, will still be found to be three to four times higher than in a nonepileptic population, matched for age with the epileptics. Lennox points to several factors that are responsible for the decline.[3] Milder forms of epilepsy are now recognized and reported. Control of seizures with antiepileptic drugs has greatly improved in the last twenty years. Previously, excessive amounts of bromides often caused mental dullness, which was mistakenly thought to be of epileptic origin, and in many cases phenobarbital had to be given in such large doses to control seizures that the patient's alertness was much reduced. The advent of Dilantin and other potent anticonvulsants, such as Mysoline® and Mesantoin, helped to change all this. With a reduction in frequency and severity of seizures, there was also a decrease in brain injury due to falls. The incidence of status epilepticus, debilitating and fatal in some cases, has been significantly lowered even among institutionalized patients. In addition, prenatal and obstetrical care and reporting have improved, and the devastating effects of many infectious diseases has been decreased. On the other hand, mentally retarded babies with congenital defects or with birth and perinatal injury, who would not have survived years ago, are now being saved and added to the list of mentally retarded potential epileptics.

Mental deficiency, when associated with epilepsy, is usually due to antecedent brain damage or to the combined effects of brain damage and epilepsy. Rarely is it due to seizures alone.

What was once called *epileptic deterioration* appears to be no different from the deterioration that occurs among patients with various types of organic brain disease with or without epilepsy. In rare cases, repeated severe convulsions (particularly status epilepticus) cause severe hypoxia and may result in deterioration. The frequency of petit mal seizures or of simple febrile convulsions bears no relationship to mental retardation.

Cases of "undifferentiated" mental retardation, in which the intellectual defect is not due to an identifiable organic brain disorder, disease, or damage, are associated with a high incidence of electroencephalographic abnormality and with clinical seizures. The types of abnormality and of clinical seizures are in general not specific for mental retardation and are essentially the same as those found among patients with identifiable organic brain disease and with epilepsy with or without mental retardation. Thus, it appears that the same abnormalities occur among mentally retarded patients who have not had seizures and those who have, and that the same type of abnormality occurs among patients who have recognized brain damage and those who have not. All of which seems to imply that important organic factors are operating in both epilepsy and in mental retardation.

The electroencephalogram does not measure intelligence; an idiot may have a normal electroencephalogram, and an exceptionally intelligent person may have a very abnormal one. There is only one electroencephalographic abnormality, namely, extreme spindles that correlates highly with mental retardation.[119] The pattern has been called *extreme spindles* because it resembles the spindles of normal sleep, but is more continuous and of higher voltage.[10] In some cases it appears even in the awake recording. It is most common in patients with cerebral palsy of the athetoid type. It presumably points to a lesion in the reticular formation. It correlates with a specific organic type of mental retardation; it is only slightly more common in cases of familial retardation than in the general population.

Retardates have a higher incidence than control subjects of abnormal fast or slow activity, indicating nonepileptic types of irritative and depressive reactions to injury. They also have generalized or focal suppression of voltage production indicating severe depressive reactions to injury and possibly destructive injuries. The paroxysmal dysrhythmias of epilepsy (i.e. various types of seizure discharge) vary in their incidence with the chronological age of the patient and not with his mental age. However, there is a general relationship between the degree of electroencephalographic abnormality, the severity of the clinical epilepsy, and the degree of intellectual subnormality.[47] Even among nonepileptic retardates, the incidence of electroencephalographic abnormality is approximately two times higher among those with severe retardation (IQ below 60) than among those with a lesser degree of retardation.

However, desirable as it might be to comfort epileptics and the parents of epileptics by insisting that epilepsy and mental retardation are unrelated, the fact is that relationships do exist between certain types of retardation and certain types of epilepsy. Infantile spasms and hypsarhythmia are highly associated with mental retardation, as is also petit mal variant. These most juvenile forms of epilepsy are the ones that are most likely to be complicated by intellectual impairment. Apparently it is the earliest injuries that are likely to result in mental retardation. Brain damage *in utero* or early infancy is more likely to be followed by mental retardation than comparable damage in childhood, adolescence, or adult life.

Chapter XXIII
CEREBRAL PALSY

Cerebral palsy, implying persistent and more or less continuous motor defects and deficits due to damage to the motor centers of the brain in childhood, is commonly complicated by mental deficiency and by epilepsy. Such patients provide examples of epilepsy associated with a great variety of different types of lesion in various parts of the brain. A study of such cases electroencephalographically[10] as well as by other methods helps not only to identify cases whose motor disability is compounded by an epileptic process, but it also helps to indicate what types of injury are most epileptogenic and to reveal the time-lag that often occurs between injury and the appearance of clinical seizures. The motor defects of cerebral palsy and the mental retardation that commonly accompanies it are chiefly due to destruction of cerebral neurons. They are associated with nonparoxysmal abnormalities in the electroencephalogram such as focal slowing or asymmetry, reduction of voltage production, and disordered sleep patterns. These findings usually accord with the type and extent of the motor disability, being bilateral in quadriplegia and unilateral in hemiplegia. The electroencephalogram is most useful when it shows paroxysmal disorder, because of nondestructive, nonlethal, irritative injuries. These usually manifest themselves in seizures, though in many cases seizure activity remains subclinical and may clear up without producing seizures. In other cases, however, seizures develop years after the seizure activity first appeared. More will be said about the predictive value of the electroencephalogram in cerebral palsy at the end of this chapter.

Different types of injury create different risks of epilepsy. Encephalitis causes the most epilepsy and the most mental retardation, and Rh incompatability, the least. As will be seen from Figure 16, the ascending rank order for the percentage incidence of seizures among cerebral palsy patients with known etiologies is as follows: Rh incompatability, prematurity, anoxia, birth trauma, and encephalitis. Thus, it appears that the earliest injuries are not (as is sometimes stated) the ones that are most highly associated with mental retardation and epilepsy.

In cerebral palsy, as in other conditions, the age of the patient at the time the electroencephalogram is recorded is an important determinant of the type of abnormality that is found (Fig. 17). In children one year of age or less, almost half (45%) have normal electroencephalograms, and hypsarhythmia is the most common electroencephalographic abnormality, but only 12 percent of patients have hypsarhythmia. With increasing age, multiple foci of spike seizure activity become the dominant abnormality. Pure petit mal and even petit mal variant are rare among patients with cerebral palsy. In Figure 17 the latter is included in the column labeled "Miscellaneous." At age four,

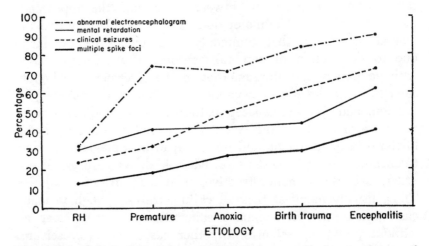

Figure 16. Relationship between the etiology and the incidence of electroencephalographic abnormality, clinical epilepsy, and mental retardation. The figure should be read as follows: 32 percent of children with cerebral palsy due to an Rh factor had abnormal electroencephalograms. (From Gibbs, F.A., and Gibbs, E.L.: *Atlas of Electroencephalography*, Reading, Massachusetts, Addison-Wesley, vol. 3, 1964.)

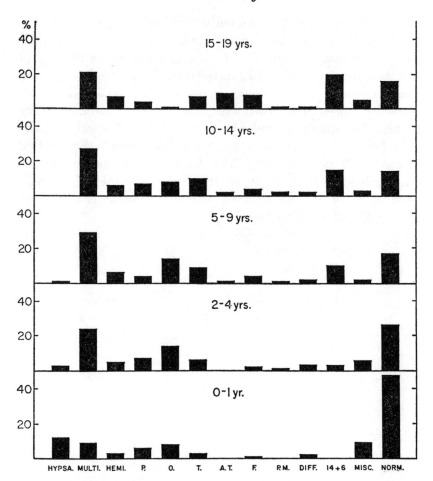

Figure 17. Electroencephalographic classification of 2,124 consecutive cases of cerebral palsy below 20 years of age. Abbreviations as follows: HYPSA.—hypsarhythmia; MULTI.—multiple foci of spikes in both hemispheres; HEMI.—widespread spike activity in one hemisphere; P., O., T., A.T., and F.—spike focus in the parietal, occipital, midtemporal, anterior temporal, and frontal areas, respectively; P.M.—3 per second spike-and-wave activity of the petit mal type; DIFF.—irregular diffuse spike-and-slow-wave discharges; 14 and 6—14 and 6 per second positive spikes, without other seizure activity; MISC.—miscellaneous abnormalities other than those listed; NORM.—normal. (From Gibbs, F.A., and Gibbs, E.L.: *Atlas of Electroencephalography*, Reading, Massachusetts, Addison-Wesley, vol. 3, 1964.)

Epilepsy Handbook

70 percent of cases of cerebral palsy have spike seizure discharges, 28 percent have spikes without clinical seizures (subclinical), and 42 percent have spikes and clinical seizures. By the age of fourteen years, 65 percent have spike discharges; only 5 percent are subclinical, and the rest, or 60 percent, have spikes with clinical seizures. A follow-up study has shown that the finding of negative spikes at any age in a child with cerebral palsy who has not had seizures creates a 50 percent chance that seizures will develop later. The finding of a normal electroencephalogram in a five-year to a nine-year old child with cerebral palsy and no seizures practically guarantees that seizures will not develop later.[10]

Chapter XXIV

GENERAL PRINCIPLES OF THERAPY

In the seizure states, the ultimate therapeutic effort should be directed toward removing whatever etiological factors or contributing causes can be identified and eliminated. Rarely in infants and young children, and almost never in adults, a metabolic defect, for example, phenylketonuria or galactosemia, is found to be responsible for the patient's seizures, and these cease when the proper corrective measures are applied. Calcium deficiency and hypoglycemia are also occasionally the cause of seizures in young children, but sometimes also in older children and adults. Seizures occurring with a febrile illness raise the possibility of encephalitis or meningitis. If the infection is bacterial, antibiotic therapy should be attempted. If the infection is viral, corticosteroids (particularly ACTH) can be tried. Virus infection of the brain is a common cause of epilepsy in children and adults. Hopefully, antiviral substances will someday become available, but at present natural immunity is all that protects us from a host of neurotropic viruses, and many persons are inadequately protected.

Often the etiological factor has ceased to operate. Even when an obvious primary cause has been removed, for example, a temporal lobe meningioma, the seizures may continue. In such cases the seizures are a chronic or late manifestation of a previous injury, a reminder that the removal of a primary cause does not necessarily reverse a pathological process once it has been initiated. In such cases the therapist is limited to symptomatic treatment. He must try to prevent the seizures or at least reduce their number or severity.

Symptomatic treatment carries a connotation of superficiality, but the physician treating an epileptic and the epileptic himself should realize that antiepileptic medication is, in a sense, substitution therapy. Antiepileptic drugs, when effective, act as a sort of chemical "patch" to cover a weak spot in a brain that is prone to develop discharges of excessive nervous energy. This "patch" holds energy release within normal bounds at critical points in the patient's brain where, because of defective local chemical processes, normal control is lacking. Thus antiepileptic drugs act as substitute regulators which meet the needs of the patient until, hopefully, the spontaneous regulation of energy release recovers. Such recovery occurs much more often than is generally supposed. (See Chapter XI.)

Many associated problems require management in epilepsy in addition to drug therapy, but in the majority of cases, the main task of the physicain is to find a drug or drugs which will reduce and limit the force of a seizure discharge so that it does not spread to become externalized in outward clinical symptoms. In a small percentage of cases it is possible to suppress the seizure discharge entirely and even to eliminate it so completely that medication can be discontinued.

Although, in general, one can predict with a certain amount of accuracy what medication will be most effective against a particular type of seizure, the medication best suited for a particular case can only be determined by trial and error, and this holds true also as regards dosage. Antiepileptic treatment must be individualized and "custom tailored." Changes of medication have to be made carefully both when the dosage is increased or decreased. Drugs are selected for trial on the basis of their safety and their efficacy, against the particular type of epilepsy from which the patient is suffering, as indicated by his history and by the electroencephalogram. (See the anticonvulsant drug chart.) The final therapeutic result depends to a considerable extent on the personal interest, the diligence, and the observational skill of the managing physician.

The safest drug that offers a reasonable prospect of success should be tried first, and the dose should be increased to tolerance as rapidly as possible. If this first drug prevents seizures, it should be retained as a maintenance medication. However, if ineffective it should be discontinued. If it is partially effective, it should be retained, and an attempt should be made to control seizures completely by the addition of supplemental doses of the next safest and generally most effective drug. The dosage of the supplementary medication should be raised to tolerance or until seizures are controlled. Complete control of seizures commonly requires a combination of drugs at the highest tolerated dosage levels. The aim should not be to use as little medication as possible, but to stop the seizures as quickly as possible with the least danger and with a minimum of side effects. By using antiepileptic substances with different side effects, it is possible to increase therapeutic power without a corresponding increase in annoying side effects.

Before starting antiepileptic medication, it is wise to require the patient to have a red blood count, a differential blood count, a serum glutamic oxaloacetic transaminase (*SGOT*) determination, and a urinalysis. Almost any drug can, in rare cases, produce blood, liver, or kidney damage, and the treating physician will be guarding himself and the patient if he has a report on the state of the blood, liver, and kidneys at the outset. In case abnormalities are present, he will want to take them into account in choosing medication and in estimating the effects of any drug that is prescribed. Further laboratory studies are necessary only in cases where untoward reactions occur or when a drug is being used that is more hazardous than most antiepileptic drugs. These are starred in the anticonvulsant drug chart, and the precautions to be taken with each are indicated.

If the suggestions for starting dosages are followed, this will allow a generally effective therapeutic level to be reached quickly. After twenty-four hours on a new drug, the patient should be required to telephone and report how he is feeling. Four days later (earlier, if disturbing symptoms have developed) he should telephone again. Monitoring the patient by phone, with the aid of an experienced secretary or clinic supervisor, is a far more efficient, expeditious, and safe way to get a patient established on new medication than fixed weekly or monthly office or clinic visits. Upward or downward adjustments in medication can be made on the doctor's orders depending on the presence or absence of side effects and on whether or not the patient reports that seizures are continuing or have ceased. If a seizure occurs after the patient has been on a certain dose of a drug for three or more days and if no troublesome side effects have occurred, the dose should be raised. If troublesome side effects have occurred, the dose should be reduced and supplemental medication added. There is no use waiting a week or a month for a drug to "take hold." As stated previously, the supplemental drug that is selected should be the one that is least toxic and most usually effective in the type of case under such consideration.

The control of epileptic disorders by chemical (pharmacological) means is still in a continuing, active phase of development. Great advances in therapeutic power may come soon, and someday an ideal drug may be discovered which will have the following characteristics:

1. Completely anticonvulsant.
2. Completely nonsedative and with no side effects at therapeutic dosage.
3. Completely nontoxic.

Such an ideal drug may sound too good to be possible, but modern pharmacology has worked miracles, and men studying this problem have specialized in doing things that were thought to be impossible. Even though an ideal drug for the treatment of epilepsy is not available, there is no shortage of proprietary and nonproprietary substances that have been found useful for treating seizure states. Table II is an inclusive list of such substances. In this long list there are many substances that are rarely used, others that are used only to treat special conditions, and still others that are not used at present or no longer being manufactured. The most useful and commonly used antiepileptic substances are illustrated in the frontispiece. In succeeding chapters, the antiepileptic substances are considered in detail in the order of their general usefulness. Most of them fall into four major groups, namely, (a) substances with a barbiturate-like

TABLE II

ANTICONVULSANT DRUGS USED IN CHILD EPILEPSY[121]

ACTH	Diuril	Peganone
Ammonium chloride	Elipsin	Phelantin
Amobarbital	Equanil	Phenobarbital
Amphetamine, Dextro	Gemonil	Phenurone
Amphetamine, Racemic	Glutamine	Prenderol
Atabrine	Hibicon	Prolixin
Aralen	Hydantal	Pyridoxine
Aureomycin	Hydantoin	Reserpine
Benadryl	Ketogenic diet	Serpasil
Benzedrine	Librium	Steroids
Bromide	Luminal	Synatan
Cardase	Mebaral	Tegretol
Celontin	Mebroin	Themisone
Conadil	Meratran	Thiantoin
Corticotropin	Mesantoin	Thorazine
Deaner	Milontin	Tranpoise
Deltoin	Miltown	Trepidone
Desoxyn	Mogadon	Tridione
Dexanyl	Mysoline	Ultran
Dexedrine	Nuvorone	Valium
Dilantin	Ospolot	Vistaril
Dimedione	Paradione	Zarontin

structure, (b) hydantoins, (c) oxazolinediones, and (d) succinimides.

L. Boshes,[120] in a discussion of the contribution of Chicago neurologists in the study and management of convulsive disorders, actually summarizes the history and salient features of many of the anticonvulsants which have been, and still are, in common usage. Elsewhere,[121] he delineates the complexities associated in the management of seizures in children.

Chapter XXV

COMMONLY EMPLOYED ANTIEPILEPTIC AGENTS

Phenobarbital

Phenobarbital heads the list of anticonvulsants because it is the safest. Clinical experience with it goes back to 1912 when Hauptmann discovered its antiepileptic properties.[122] Except for bromides,[123,124] it is the oldest of the anticonvulsants. It has three disadvantages: (a) it is not a powerful antiepileptic drug; (b) it is a sedative, and it commonly causes drowsiness at therapeutic dosage; and (c) in children, particularly those who are hyperactive or brain damaged, it commonly causes paradoxical excitement (irritability and motor restlessness). Phenobarbital can be employed in young children and also in adults when the life situation permits a trial of minimal medication. However, before prescribing such medication for adults, the physician should remember that a single seizure can be catastrophic; it may seriously impair a patient's earning power, his social standing, and his self-confidence.

Phenobarbital is used to best advantage to supplement the more potent anticonvulsant action of Dilantin. If phenobarbital is given to an adult at bedtime in a dosage of 100 mg, it usually does not cause significant daytime drowsiness, and it provides maximum protection during sleep. This is important, for in many cases, it is during sleep that seizures are most likely to occur.

There is no reason to fear that an epileptic patient for whom phenobarbital has been prescribed will become a "barbiturate addict." This drug is not truly habit forming. Barbiturate addicts probably have some character defect that is entirely unrelated to epilepsy. They rarely use phenobarbital, preferring other barbiturates, such as Seconal® and Nembutal®. Phenobarbital addiction, if it occurs at all among epileptics, must be exceedingly rare; almost all patients want to reduce rather than increase their barbiturate intake.

The chief hazard with phenobarbital is not its use, but its sudden discontinuation. If phenobarbital medication is abruptly stopped, seizures are likely to be precipitated (withdrawal convulsions). These can be avoided if the dose is reduced gradually over a period of at least five days.

A good starting dose of phenobarbital is 100 mg at bedtime for adults and 50 mg for children. If this does not result in control of seizures, the bedtime dose can be increased provided the patient is not too drowsy on arising. Additional doses can be given during the day. Tablets of 30 mg for adults and 15 mg for children are convenient for establishing the maximal tolerated dose.

Manufacturer—Many companies

Preparations —15–30–60–100 mg tablets
15 mg per teaspoon, elixir
60–120 mg ampules for parenteral use (IV or IM)

Dilantin Sodium (United States) Epineutin (Britain) (Diphenylhydantoin)

Dilantin is a powerful nonsedative antiepileptic drug of low toxicity.[125,126] It has a broad range of action against many types of seizure, and though it is relatively ineffective against petit mal seizures associated with three per second spike-and-wave discharges, it may in some cases prevent such seizures. Not uncommonly, however, it flares up petit mal disorder. It is the most generally useful of all antiepilepitc medications and is the drug of choice in all types of epilepsy. Even in cases of petit mal, particularly when complicated by grand mal, it is worth trying. If a flare-up of petit mal seizures occurs, no harm will be done, provided the parents are prepared for this eventuality. Dilantin can be discontinued or the dose reduced and other more specific antipetit mal medication prescribed.

Most older children and adults experience no annoying side effects when taking 100 mg of this drug three times a day with meals. A dose of 30 mg three times a day with meals usually causes no side effects in children. These should not be considered standard doses. The dose should be raised to tolerance, i.e. adjusted by trial to a little less than that which produces disturbing side effects. Dilantin, in rare and atypical cases, causes drowsiness. Its usual limiting side effects are dizziness and double vision. Motor incoordination may develop with staggering and nystagmus. Other important toxic reactions include gingival hyperplasia, hirsutism, a measles-like rash with fever, tremor, a cerebellar-like syndrome, and a lymphoma-like picture. Such symptoms are not usually evidence of dangerous intoxication; they usually diminish within a few days when the dosage is lowered and clear up entirely in a week or so when the Dilantin is discontinued. In some cases, Dilantin causes gastric irritation, but this may be avoided or minimized by taking the drug before, during, or after meals or by taking it in coated capsules.

Dilantin-induced hyperplasia of the gums, mentioned above, occurs in about 20 percent of children;[126] it does not occur in adults. It is an idiosyncratic reaction and not due to vitamin deficiency. Although inconvenient and sometimes painful and certainly disfiguring, especially in a girl, it disappears or becomes less marked if Dilantin medication is discontinued, and it may subside to a tolerable level if the dosage is reduced. Often there is a hygienic factor associated with it.[127] It can be retarded by good mouth hygiene and by massage of the gums. Even when overgrowth is extreme, if Dilantin controls the seizures better than any other drug, the patient may continue with this medication and have the excess gum tissue removed periodically by a competent oral surgeon, rather than relinquish the protective action of the Dilantin. Overgrowth of body hair occurs in a small percentage of people taking Dilantin; if seriously disfiguring or embarrassing, the patient should be changed to some other type of anticonvulsant medication. About 2 percent of people are sensitive to this drug, reacting with a blotchy, measles-like rash often associated with a high fever. In such a case, the Dilantin should be discontinued at once and the patient placed on phenobarbital. Of course, if an extremely rare case is encountered in which a hemorrhagic reaction develops or there are severe cerebellar symptoms, the Dilantin should be stopped immediately. When mild reactions have occurred, medication with Dilantin can be gradually and cautiously reinstated once the reaction has subsided, provided blood, liver, and kidney tests are normal.

The usual starting dose of Dilantin for adults is 100 mg three times a day with meals, and for children, 30 mg administered in the same manner.[128]

Manufacturer—Parke Davis

Preparations — 50 mg Infatabs
              30 and 100 mg capsules
              100 mg per teaspoon, suspension
              100 mg delayed action capsules (D.A.)
              Parenteral 50 mg/cc

Mysoline® (United States) Primidone (Britain) (5-Phenyl-5-Ethyl-Hexahydropyrimadine-4-6 Dione)

Mysoline[129,130] has been used for a long enough time and in a sufficient number of cases to show that it is a useful antiepileptic substance of low toxicity. Drowsiness is the most usual limiting side effect. The sleepiness, which is especially common when Mysoline medication is first started, usually disappears at the end of one month. (See Stimulants in Chapter XXVI.) However, if Mysoline is started in a low dosage of 50 mg and increased gradually, the somnifacient effect is not so troublesome. However, one must be prepared to find occasional patients who are extremely sensitive to Mysoline, who sleep for eighteen hours even on small doses. If phenobarbital was used as a previous anticonvulsant medication, it is advisable to reduce it gradually as the Mysoline is raised, because it adds to the soporific effect of the Mysoline and usually interferes with the attainment of a maximally effective Mysoline dosage.

A few patients on Mysoline develop a diffuse measles-like rash. Occasionally in psychomotor epilepsy this drug may precipitate an acute psychosis-like reaction, but in this respect it is not different from a number of other antiepileptic substances. Rarely has any damage been reported to the blood, liver, or kidneys. Occasionally a transient leukopenia may be observed, but whether this is due to the Mysoline is questionable. Sometimes ataxia, dizziness, irritability, anorexia, nausea and vomiting, edema, or sexual impotence are reported, but these, if causally related to the Mysoline, subside with decreased dosage or discontinuation of this form of medication.

Usually Mysoline is started by adding a 50 mg tablet at bedtime to whatever other anticonvulsant the patient is taking. If this is well tolerated, the dose is increased to two 50 mg tablets at bedtime. The next step might be to shift to one half of the 250 mg tablet or go up in steps, using 50 mg tablets and shifting later to whole 250 mg tablets, the aim being to increase the dosage until seizures are controlled or handicapping side effects develop.[130]

Manufacturer—Ayerst

Preparations — 50 mg tablets
                 250 mg tablets
                 125 mg flavored tablet (in Canada)
                 250 mg per teaspoon, suspension

Mesantoin (Methylphenylethyl Hydantoin)

When seizures do not respond to Dilantin, or Dilantin and phenobarbital, or to Dilantin and Mysoline in combination, and if they are not of the petit mal type, maximal tolerated doses of Mesantoin should be tried.[131,132] This medication should be added to whatever Dilantin and phenobarbital or Dilantin and Mysoline dosages have been found most advantageous for the patient, but the phenobarbital and Mysoline dosages should be lowered as the Mesantoin dosage is raised. Mesantoin commonly produces drowsiness, and the sedative action of all these drugs is additive. (See "Stimulants" in Chapter XXVI.)

Since Mesantoin does not produce hyperplasia of the gums, it can be used to replace Dilantin in cases where the latter has caused this unpleasant side effect. Roughly 10 percent of patients are sensitive to Mesantoin regardless of the rate at which the dosage is increased. This sensitivity usually manifests itself within a week or two after the beginning of Mesantoin therapy by one or more of the following symptoms: fever, lymphadenopathy (usually most evident at the base of the scalp or in the neck), and a scarlatiniform or morbiliform rash (usually most evident over the chest or upper portions of the back). This skin reaction is sometimes difficult to distinguish from that seen in scarlet fever or measles. When the rash is absent, but when the cervical glands are enlarged, the appearance of the patient, his blood count, or even the histological changes found at a biopsy may lead to an erroneous diagnosis of Hodgkin's disease.

If Mesantoin is continued in the face of a sensitivity reaction, serious blood damage may result. However, if the drug is discontinued quickly, the entire reaction usually reverses without the development of a serious blood dyscrasia.[133]

It must be remembered that in highly sensitive individuals, bone marrow damage may occur without warning. This fortunately is rare, but it is one of the truly dangerous features of this drug. However, if Mesantoin is reserved for severe, resistant cases, this danger can be accepted as a calculated risk. If the reaction continues, is mild, and the blood picture is unchanged, Mesantoin therapy can be cautiously and gradually started again when the reaction has subsided.[134]

Any patient on Mesantoin should have regular blood counts, blood-platelet estimations, liver function tests, such as SGOT (serum glutamic oxaloacetic transaminase) determinations, on a routine basis before starting Mesantoin, two weeks later, and monthly thereafter.[135] If the leukocyte count drops below 4,000 or if there is a sudden or marked drop in the neutrophils (below 40%), daily blood counts are advisable for a few days. If the absolute number of neutrophils per cubic millimeter (white blood count multiplied by percent of neutrophils in the differential count) drops to 1,500, the Mesantoin should be stopped. The patient should be told that a small percentage of patients on this drug have untoward reactions and that they should report at once any new signs or symptoms.

The starting dose of Mesantoin for adults is 100 mg at bedtime, and for children, 50 mg (half of the scored tablet) or less, depending on the age and weight of the child. As with other antiepileptic drugs, the dose should be individualized by increasing in steps of 50 mg every five days until troublesome side effects develop and then, by reducing the dose to one that is well tolerated.

Manufacturer—Sandoz

Preparations —100 mg tablets

Tridione® (Trimethadione or Trimethyloxyzolidine Dione)

Tridione eliminates seizures or greatly reduces their frequency in approximately 83 percent of patients with petit mal.[136,137] In rare instances, Tridione and, also, Paradione® (like most other antiepileptic substances) may normalize the electroencephalogram, but usually the clinical response is greater than the electroencephalographic responses and, as with other antiepileptic substances, the clinical seizures may cease even though interseizure discharges continue unaltered. If the seizures have been controlled with Tridione (or some other type of medication) and if the electroencephalogram has become normal both awake and asleep, the Tridione (or other medication) can usually be reduced or omitted without recurrence of seizures.

Tridione in a high percentage of cases increases grand mal seizures, if these are present. The finding of a strong grand mal component (multiple spikes) in the electroencephalogram in a case with seizures of the petit mal type raises the possibility that when the patient is placed on Tridione, the grand mal disorder will be intensified. If tonic-clonic convulsions have not occurred previously in such a case, Tridione may precipitate the patient's first grand mal seizure, and the physician may be accused of having made the patient a "true epileptic." Of course, this is a misinterpretation, for the patient already had seizures and must have had grand mal disorder; otherwise the Tridione would not have precipitated a convulsion. Discontinuation of Tridione will restore the patient to his previous state, but will not guarantee that he will not subsequently have recurring clinical seizures of the grand mal type.[136,137]

As already mentioned in the section dealing with Dilantin, this drug increases petit mal seizures in some patients. Tridione and Dilantin used in combination for treatment of cases having both grand mal and petit mal may be effective, but often they are not. In many cases, these two drugs seem to neutralize each other's therapeutic effects.

Phenobarbital or Mysoline may be added to Tridione in cases where there is a combination of grand mal and petit mal. Although phenobarbital and Mysoline have no significant anti-petit mal action, neither do they, like Dilantin, tend to precipitate seizures of the petit mal type, and both have an antigrand mal action. The difficulty of using Mysoline, phenobarbital, and Tridione together arises from the fact that each causes somnolence, and a sufficient antipetit mal and antigrand mal action usually cannot be obtained without hypersomnia. (See Stimulants in next chapter.)

A common limiting side effect of Tridione is a sensitivity to bright light called day blindness or hemeralopia.[136] It is less common in children than in adults. The patient may complain that "it looks as though it is snowing" when he goes outdoors, or he may state that "everything looks hazy" in a brightly lighted room. In order to prevent seizures and in hope of later reducing the dosage, it might be wise to exceed temporarily a comfortable level of Tridione medication. Sometimes the patient may become adjusted to a degree of hemeralopia that at the outset is very disturbing, or the hemeralopia may de-

crease even though the dosage is maintained. Generally hemeralopia subsides within a few days to a week after the Tridione
is discontinued. Sometimes the simple expedient of wearing a
pair of dark glasses takes care of the entire problem. In some
cases, drowsiness and irritability are annoying side effects of
this drug.

An acneform rash and, occasionally, cutaneous abscesses on
the face also occur as a sensitivity reaction to Tridione. A more
serious reaction, which may be asymptomatic until it has gone
too far to be reversed, is the wholesale destruction of white
cells and blood platelets. Several cases of fatal blood damage
have been reported.[138] A blood profile is recommended before
starting Tridione to determine whether the count is normal at the
onset. Patients on this drug should have a blood count, platelet
estimation, SGOT (serum glutamic oxaloacetic transaminase)
determination, and urinalysis at the start of treatment, two
weeks later, and monthly thereafter. As with other drugs that
have produced fatalities, the patient and his family should be
warned that a few patients are sensitive to Tridione and that
they should report any untoward developments at once. If the
leukocyte count drops below 4,000, or if there is a marked drop
in neutrophils below 40 percent, daily blood counts are advisable
for a few days. If the absolute number of neutrophils per cubic
millimeter (the white blood count multiplied by the percent
of neutrophils in the differential count) drops to 1,500, the
Tridione should be stopped. The neutrophil count usually returns to normal within a few weeks, but once a sensitivity to
Tridione has been found, it usually is not wise to reinstitute
Tridione therapy.

Combined medication with Tridione and Mesantoin is not
particularly effective in cases of combined petit mal and grand
mal. It is hazardous to use these two drugs in combination because both can produce blood damage. This combination should
be avoided if the seizures can be controlled by any other
means.[139]

A good initial dosage of Tridione is 300 mg TID, and children
under 2 years of age should start with 150 mg TID. The dosage
should be increased every three to four days until seizures are

completely controlled or until disturbing side effects develop. It may be necessary to increase the adult dosage up to 6 capsules daily.

Manufacturer—Abbott

Preparations —300 mg capsules
150 mg tablets Dulcets
150 mg per teaspoon solution

Paradione (Methyloxyzolidine Dione) (Paramethadione)

Paradione is a useful drug for the treatment of petit mal seizures, absences, akinetic, and myoclonic attacks.[2] In general, it has antipetit mal action equal to or slightly less than that of Tridione.[138] But in some cases it is effective when Tridione is ineffective. Like Tridione, Paradione can precipitate grand mal seizures in susceptible persons, and it also has been reported to have caused blood damage, hepatitis, and a nephrotic syndrome. Visual disturbances, hemeralopia, or "glare phenomenon" are fairly common. Other side effects (with the exception of somnolence) are less common than with Tridione. However, drowsiness, ataxia, tremor, diplopia, and a rash have been reported in patients taking Paradione.[135,138]

Paradione is usually started at a dosage of 300 mg three times a day for adults and 150 mg four times a day for children. In some adults the dosage must be increased to 3 gm per day (10 of the 300 mg capsules) before the patient's seizures are brought under control. Sometimes, when this has been accomplished, the dose can be gradually reduced without a recurrence of seizures.

Manufacturer—Abbott

Preparations —150 mg capsules
300 mg capsules
300 mg/cc, solution

Celontin® (Methsuximide)

Celontin is closely related chemically to Milontin® and Zarontin®. (See next section.) It is useful for the treatment of petit mal and particularly valuable in mixed cases of grand mal and petit mal because it does not "trigger" grand mal seizures.[140] It is also valuable in some cases of grand mal and of psychomotor epilepsy,[146] and it may eliminate seizures in highly resistant cases when added as a third drug to supplement a combination of Dilantin and Mysoline or Dilantin and Mesantoin.

The most usual side effects are drowsiness, ataxia, anorexia, nausea, and vomiting. A rash occurs in some cases. Side effects and any toxic reactions that develop usually disappear promptly when Celontin is discontinued. If drowsiness is the only side effect, it may be helped if some of the other anticonvulsants being employed with Celontin are reduced. A few cases of leukopenia, which cleared up when the Celontin was discontinued, have been reported.[141]

One capsule of Celontin (150 or 300 mgs) can be used as a starting dose or added to whatever other medication the patient is taking. Dosage should be gradually increased until seizures cease or until limiting side effects develop.

Manufacturer—Parke-Davis

Preparations —150 mg capsules
                300 mg capsules

Zarontin (Ethosuximide)

Zarontin is highly effective against petit mal, absences, akinetic, and myoclonic seizures, especially when these are associated with three per second spike-and-wave discharges in the electroencephalogram.[142] In general it is no more toxic than Milontin or Celontin, but it commonly produces drowsiness, dizziness, nausea, vomiting, and diarrhea. It can produce a skin rash and blood disturbances, and a few cases of pancytopenia have been reported.

Zarontin has a strong antipetit mal and a weak antigrand mal and antipsychomotor action. In some cases, it is more effective than Celontin or Milontin or any other substance.[143,144]

This drug may be started with one-half to one tablet one to two times a day.

Manufacturer—Parke-Davis

Preparations —250 mg tablets

Milontin (Phensuximide)

Milontin has significant antipetit mal action,[145,146] but in general it is not as potent as Tridione, Paradione, Zarontin, or Celontin. It commonly produces headache, somnolence, nausea, vomiting, and dizziness, and rarely, a rash with accompanying fever.

Manufacturer—Parke-Davis

Preparations —500 mg capsules
                250 mg per teaspoon, suspension

Phenurone® (Phenacemide-Phenacetylcarbamide)

Phenurone is effective against grand mal, petit mal, and even psychomotor seizures. It is the first, and so far the most potent general antiepileptic substance that has been developed. Although it rarely produces somnolence or other handicapping side effects at a therapeutically effective dosage and although it is generally a nontoxic substance, about four persons in one thousand react to it with serious liver damage.[147-150] Patients receiving this drug should have Ehrlich's quantitative urinary urobilinogen test (by the method of Wallace and Diamond) performed monthly. A positive reaction for urobilinogen in dilutions of urine above 1:20 should be followed immediately by more precise liver function studies, such as bromsulfalein dye retention, icteric index, cephalin flocculation, thymol turbidity, and a serum glutamic oxaloacetic transaminase (SGOT) estimation. If these results indicate liver damage, Phenurone should be discontinued immediately. The prescribing physician should also be on the alert for and should warn against signs of liver dysfunction, such as jaundice, flatulence, weight loss, weakness, or other signs of ill health. When these directions are followed, the hazard of serious irreversible liver damage is greatly reduced, but it cannot be entirely eliminated. It is doubtful that Phenurone alone can produce blood dyscrasia or kidney damage. Nevertheless, as a wise precaution, when the patient visits the laboratory for his monthly urobilinogen test, he might ask for the full battery of tests that are commonly used to pick up evidence of toxic effects on blood-forming organs, the liver, and the kidney. These, as indicated in previous sections, are the following: (a) a complete blood count, including a blood platelet estimation, (b) an SGOT (serum glutamic oxaloacetic transaminase) determination, and (c) a urinalysis.

Since Phenurone is used in cases which are resistant to anticonvulsant medications, it is used most commonly in cases with psychomotor seizures, in those with a combination of grand mal and petit mal, and those with persistent, severely handicapping types of seizure. In such cases it may produce what seems like a miraculous elimination of seizures. The effect is most dramatic when a person who is having hundreds of petit mal, akinetic seizures, or other types of minor seizures per day, in spite of maximal and even supramaximal tolerated dosage of all other antiepileptic drugs, suddenly becomes seizure-free and to all appearances seems to be well soon after being started on Phenurone.

This drug produces complete or marked control of seizures in 50 percent of patients with psychomotor seizures, who are refractory to other medications.[147] In such patients, however, Phenurone tends to exacerbate the psychiatric disorder that is commonly present. This unfortunate complication occasionally occurs with other drugs, but it is more usual with Phenurone. The patient's relatives must be warned that if new psychiatric symptoms appear or old ones increase, this may be a drug effect, and they should notify the doctor immediately. Patients who have not had personality disturbances rarely develop psychiatric symptoms on Phenurone, and in such cases it can be used with less hesitation. Phenurone does not produce a peculiar kind of psychiatric disorder. As a rule, it merely intensifies the kind of psychiatric disorder from which the patient previously suffered; such disorders usually subside promptly when Phenurone is discontinued.[151]

The amount of Phenurone that is necessary to prevent seizures determines the dosage, and this must be individualized for each patient. One tablet of 500 mg three times a day, added to the patient's current antiepileptic medications, is a good starting dose. The dose may be increased gradually by adding one tablet every four days until seizures are controlled or until annoying side effects develop. However, ten tablets a day, a total of 5 gm, is the maximum dose. When seizures are controlled for several months, medication may be simplified and improved by slowly reducing other anticonvulsants that may be producing disturbing or annoying side effects and that may be no longer needed for seizure control.

Manufacturer—Abbott

Preparations —300 mg (enteric coated) tablets
500 mg tablets

Mebaral® (Mephobarbital)

The indications for Mebaral are the same as those for phenobarbital. In cases with a combination of grand mal and petit mal, Mebaral is often useful[152] because it has a slight antipetit mal action and provides some protection against grand mal. Although its antipetit mal and antigrand mal actions are both weak, it does not seem to precipitate either type of disorder and therefore may be used in combination with Tridione or Paradione to decrease their convulsant effect in predisposed persons and to add slightly to the total antipetit mal action. The effective dose of this drug is usually twice that of phenobarbital.

The starting dose is 30 mg once or twice a day.

Manufacturer—Winthrop

Preparations — 30 mg tablets
50 mg tablets
100 mg tablets

Gemonil® (Metharbital)

Gemonil has less sedative action than phenobarbital, and it has been reported[153] to be particularly effective in the "organic type of petit mal" associated with myoclonic seizures[154] and major convulsions and with neurological deficits (i.e. petit mal variant).

The usual limiting side effects are drowsiness, ataxia, and occasionally irritability.

The starting dose for adults is 100 mg once or twice daily, and for children, one-fourth to one-half of the 100 mg tablet once or twice daily.

Manufacturer—Abbott

Preparations —100 mg tablets

Peganone® (3-Ethyl 5-Phenylhydantoin Ethotoin)

Peganone was developed as a low-potency, antiepileptic hydantoin in an effort to avoid the limiting side effects of other hydantoins while still retaining useful anticonvulsant action.[155] It is relatively nontoxic and, unlike Dilantin, does not produce gingival hyperplasia or hirsutism. When added to other antiepileptic drugs, it sometimes adds just enough antiepileptic power to eliminate seizures entirely. The usual limiting side effects are somnolence, ataxia, and gastric disturbances. In some patients it produces a rash.[156]

Though this drug is relatively nontoxic, careful watch must still be kept for signs and symptoms of blood, liver, or kidney damage, and appropriate laboratory studies promptly instituted.

Peganone in general is more effective in grand mal than in other types of epilepsy. In some cases it has been used to control psychomotor seizures. Its chief value is to supplement other antiepileptic medication. If other drugs control seizures, but produce unpleasant side effects in the required dosages, Peganone can sometimes be added and the dosage of the original medication reduced to a more tolerable level.

Patients may be started on one or two 250 mg tablets daily.

Manufacturer—Abbott

Preparations —250 mg tablets
             500 mg tablets

Chapter XXVI

ACCESSORY DRUGS EMPLOYED

Librium® (Chlordiazepoxide)

Librium is sometimes of value in mixed types of epilepsy, but in general it is less effective than Valium®. It is most useful as a mild tranquilizer for children with epilepsy complicated by behavior disturbances.

Starting dosage for adults is 5 mg three times a day, and for children, 5 mg twice a day. The dose should be individualized and raised until seizures are controlled or limiting side effects develop. The most usual side effects are somnolence and ataxia.[2,156-158]

Manufacturer—Roche

Preparations —5–10–25 mg capsules

Valium (Diazepam)

Valium is particularly indicated in the management of status epilepticus and seems almost specific.[159-162] There are dangers in the use of this drug because of a synergistic action of barbiturates with diazepam.[162]

It is also known to be efficacious in status epilepticus of the petit mal variety. Valium may also be effective in the control of seizure activity resulting from an acute brain insult.

Toxicity consists of drowsiness, ataxia, diplopia, incoordination, vertigo, and rarely, a rash.

Manufacturer—Roche

Preparations —2–5–10 mg tablets
2 cc ampules containing 10 mg of the drug

Tegretol® (Carbamazepine)

This drug is related to the phenothiazines and is particularly valuable in the management of tic douloureux or of intractable headaches[163] and other facial pain.[164]

Early reports indicate favorable results in the management of some patients with grand mal and psychomotor seizures.[165,166] Limiting side effects are drowsiness, blurring of vision, headache, nausea, vomiting, irritability, and ataxia. This drug can produce agranulocytosis, kidney and liver damage, hypotension, peripheral neuritis, and depression.

Manufacturer—Geigy
Preparation —200 mg tablets

Mogadon® (Nitrazepam)

Mogadon is particularly useful for patients with infantile spasms and myoclonic seizures in early childhood.[167-170] Unlike ACTH, Mogadon does not normalize the electroencephalogram, nor does it help to avoid the intellectual defects that are so likely to occur in patients with hypsarhythmia and infantile spasms. In some patients with other types of seizures it is dramatically effective when nothing else helps. It is an analogue of Librium, but in the cases where it is effective, it is more potent than Librium or Valium. In some cases it increases grand mal seizures and has to be discontinued, but in others, additional anticonvulsant medication leads to a satisfactory result with reduction or elimination of all epileptic manifestations. Unfortunately, in spite of the fact that Mogadon has been used in Europe for many years, the drug is still classified in the United States as an experimental drug by the Pure Food and Drug Administration.

Side effects include the following: drowsiness, ataxia, irritability, muscular hypotonia, anorexia, nausea, vomiting, and skin rash. The starting dose for adults is 5 to 10 mg three times a day, and for infants to one year, 1 mg three times a day, increasing to 2 mg.

Manufacturer—Hoffman—La Roche
Preparation —2–5–10 mg tablets

ACTH and Corticosteroids

Both ACTH and corticosteroids have been used, particularly in children, not only to reduce or eliminate seizures, but also to improve the electroencephalographic tracing. ACTH is especially effective for the treatment of hypsarhythmia and infantile spasms.[173-178] However, good results are obtained in a high percentage of cases only when maximal doses of ACTH are used. Newborn infants and those up to two months of age should be given 20 units per day. Babies, three to six months of age, should be given 40 units per day. Children six months of age to one year should be given 80 units per day, and those over one year, 120 units.[179] These may sound like high doses, but if low doses are used at the outset, there appears to be a tendency for the child to become resistant to ACTH. If one or both parents are sufficiently intelligent, the necessary daily intramuscular injections can be given by a parent after she or he has been instructed by a doctor or nurse. Some patients respond well to Pregnisone®,[150] and of course oral administration simplifies treatment, but ACTH is the drug of choice. In general, children with hypsarhythmia tolerate ACTH exceptionally well. The aim should be to normalize the electroencephalogram as quickly as possible.

As long as clinical seizures continue, hypsarhythmia will be present, but the electroencephalogram is useful for monitoring the response to treatment even in the presence of a seizure. A decrease in seizure activity is a good prognostic sign. However, discontinuation of ACTH treatment because clinical seizures have ceased and because the waking electroencephalogram has become normal is risky; the sleep tracing may still show hypsarhythmia, and if so, a relapse is likely. Treatment should be continued until hypsarhythmia is no longer present in the sleep recording or until it has become clear that maximum, tolerated doses of ACTH are ineffective. Before abandoning ACTH treatment entirely, a final effort should be made with intravenous ACTH.

ACTH has also been shown to be effective in other forms of juvenile epilepsy.[176] However, it does not have value in adult forms of epilepsy.[173] Long term results with the treatment of petit mal are generally unsatisfactory. Almost everyone who has

136 *Epilepsy Handbook*

studied the matter seriously agrees that ACTH is relatively specific for infantile spasms associated with hypsarhythmia.

Manufacturer—Many companies

Preparations —Both oral and parenteral

Diamox® (Acetazolamide)

Diamox is a sulfonamide derivative which has an inhibitory effect on the carbonic anhydrase enzyme system. It was introduced as a diuretic for congestive heart failure and for renal disease, and this remains its major area of usefulness. Its therapeutic power in petit mal is probably related to its ability to block the normal pathway of carbon dioxide transport. High CO_2 tension raises, and low CO_2 tension lowers the petit mal threshold. Diamox has none of the toxic properties of the sulfonamides. It has considerable therapeutic efficacy in petit mal epilepsy.[150,171,172,180,181]

Because of its low toxicity, as compared with Tridione and Paradione, Celontin, Zarontin, or Phenurone, it might be tried first, before any of them. Usually, however, it is not powerful enough to suppress petit mal seizures when used alone. Its greatest usefulness is as an adjunct to other antipetit mal substances.[182]

For children, one-half tablet (125 mg) twice daily is a good initial dose. It may be increased to three to four tablets a day depending upon control of seizures or the occurrence of side effects, such as loss of appetite, acidosis, numbness, drowsiness, ataxia, nausea, and urinary incontinence. An adult may start with a whole tablet twice a day and may increase to six tablets a day.

Manufacturer—Lederle

Preparations —250 mg tablets
500 mg ampules, IM or IV

Stimulants

Caffeine may be used to antagonize the soporific effect of some of the antiepileptic drugs. This can be done without seriously affecting the anticonvulsant activity of the original drug. Caffeine is sometimes effective in controlling myoclonic seizures and may be helpful in treating petit mal.[183] Limiting side effects are sleeplessness and a feeling of jitteryness.

The starting dose for caffeine is 7.5 gm for adults and one-half of the dose for children.

Dexedrine® (Dextroamphetamine)

The indications for the use of Dexedrine are roughly the same as those for Desoxyn® and Benzedrine®; their toxicity is also the same. However, the dextro-rotatory form of amphetamine, i.e. Dexedrine, is sometimes more effective and generally produces fewer side effects than other drugs with a similar stimulating action. It may be useful in patients with seizures[2] and/or behavior disorders, and it can be used to counteract the soporific effect of antiepileptic substances.

The starting dose for adults is 5 mg, and for children, 2.5 mg. The dose should be raised until symptoms are controlled or disturbing side effects, such as insomnia, increased excitability, or restlessness, develop.

Manufacturer—Smith Kline and French

Preparation   —Tablets, 5, 10, 15 mg
        Elixir, 5 cc, 5 mg
        Spansules, 5, 10, 15 mg

Desoxyn (Methamphetamine Hydrochloride)

This drug seems efficacious, particularly in the absence of akinetic attacks. It is also used as a drug to counteract the somnorific effect of the anticonvulsants, and is especially effective in narcolepsy.[2]

There is some toxicity to include insomnia, irritability, anorexia, and even weight loss.

Manufacturer—Abbott

Preparations   —2.5 mg tablets
        5 mg tablets
        5–10–15 mg gradumets
        2–5 mg to a teaspoon of the elixir

Aralen® (Chloroquine) Atabrine® (Quinacrine)

Aralen and Atabrine have been shown to have an antipetit mal action,[184] and they have been used successfully to treat petit mal status.[2] However, they may exacerbate grand mal seizures in patients who have both petit mal and grand mal.

Unpleasant side effects include yellow discoloration of the skin, as well as nausea, vomiting, abdominal pain, diarrhea, and other signs and symptoms of liver disturbance.

Manufacturer—Winthrop

Preparations —250 mg ampules
125 mg ampules

Miscellaneous Drugs of the "Tranquilizer" Group

Meprobamate (Miltown® or Equanil®)

Now and then reports appear of the benefits of meprobamate in the management of epilepsy. The consensus, however, is that this drug does not contribute significantly to the control of seizures.[2,185]

Manufacturer—Wallace (Miltown®)

Preparation —Miltown 200 mg and 400 mg tablets
Meprospan 400 mg capsules
Meprotabs 400 mg

Manufacturer—Wyeth (Equanil®)

Preparation —200 mg-400 mg tablets
400 mg release capsules

Mellaril® (Thioridazine)

Manufacturer—Sandoz

Preparation —10, 25, 50, 200 mg tablets

Thorazine® (Chlorpromazine)

Manufacturer—Smith Kline and French

Preparation —Tablets, 10, 25, 50, 75, 100 mg
Liquid concentrate, 30 mg/cc
Suppositories, 25, 100 mg
Spansules, 30, 75, 150, 200 mg
Vials, 10 cc (25 mg) 10 cc, 25 mg/cc—parenteral use
Ampules, 1–25 cc, 25 mg/cc

Vesprin® (Triflupromazine)

Manufacturer—Squibb

Preparation —Vesprin injection 10 mg/cc—10 cc vial
20 mg/cc—10 cc vial

Stelazine® (Brand Trifluoperazine)

Manufacturer—Smith Kline and French

Preparation —Tablets, 1 and 2 mg

Serpasil® (Reserpine)

Manufacturer—Ciba
Preparation —Tablets, 0.25 mg, 0.1 mg, 1.0 mg
Elixir, 0.2 mg/4ml
Ampules, 2 ml/cc—parenteral

Bromides

In some cases bromides control seizures[123,124] when nothing else does. However, bromides, though they were the first anticonvulsant to be discovered, are not in general use because the toxic and anticonvulsant doses are almost the same. At an effective anticonvulsant dosage they commonly produce lethargy, somnolence, and confusion. In young people bromides often cause an acneform eruption, which sometimes results in disfiguring scars. In adults they can cause a toxic psychosis. The dosage is hard to regulate if the patient's sodium chloride intake is not controlled. (Sodium chloride tends to drive out the bromide salts, and bromides accumulate when chlorides are reduced.) Therefore, the patient's diet should contain fairly constant amounts of sodium chloride. In hot weather, however, the salt intake must be increased to compensate for loss of sodium chloride through perspiration. Gastrointestinal disturbances are common among patients on bromides. If the blood level of bromide exceeds that which is safe (75–100 mg per 100 ml), it can be reduced by giving the patient sodium chloride and diuretics.

Manufacturers —many drug companies

Preparation   —sodium or potassium bromide
   15 mg tablet
   15 mg per teaspoon, elixir

Ketogenic Diet

Before the advent of Tridione, the ketogenic diet[186] was commonly employed in the management of petit mal epilepsy. Its therapeutic effect presumably depends upon a shift of the body metabolism toward acidosis.[187] In children under eight years of age, this is relatively easy to accomplish, and the ketogenic diet often leads to a cessation of seizures or to a significant reduction in their number. In older children, however, a ketosis is more difficult to obtain, and the diet is less effective.

The ketogenic diet, as ordinarily used, includes a large amount of fat and a moderate amount of protein and excludes carbohydrates and starches. This diet is expensive, troublesome to obtain and prepare, and children commonly find it distasteful. In most cases, it turns out to be impractical even when beneficial, but it is demonstrably effective in a significant number of cases of petit mal and can be used as a supplement to Tridione and/or Paradione in the treatment of petit mal.

Chapter XXVII

SURGICAL TREATMENT

Patients with epilepsy whose seizures cannot be prevented with medication and whose seizures are seriously handicapping should be considered for neurosurgical treatment.[33,188] If a consistent unilateral, clearly defined focus can be demonstrated preoperatively in the electroencephalogram or if definite clinical signs of localized disorder are present, the case may be one that is favorable for exploration and possibly for surgical removal of the focus. The evaluation of patients for surgery and the surgical treatment of suitable patients, as well as their postoperative care, should be delegated to a surgeon or a group of surgeons with special interest and special competence in the removal of epileptogenic lesions.

The following is a summary of the indications for surgical treatment of epilepsy:

1. Seriously handicapping epileptic seizures that cannot be prevented by any antiepileptic drugs at tolerable dosage.
2. A consistent focus of seizure activity awake and asleep.
3. Clinical seizures according with the focus of the electroencephalographic seizure discharge.
4. No great likelihood of improvement with increasing age.
5. The area implicated by the electroencephalographic discharge and by the clinical signs and symptoms must be one which, if attacked surgically, will not leave the patient with a serious speech defect or an overwhelming neurological deficit.
6. The chance of a good therapeutic result will be increased if there is evidence of a structural lesion in the same area as the epileptic focus.
7. The overall therapeutic value of surgical treatment is

greatly affected by the intellectual and mental status of the patient. Surgery does not offer hope of rehabilitation to epileptics who are severely retarded or psychotic. However, if psychiatric symptoms are present, the question of whether they constitute an indication for or against surgery should be decided by the neurosurgeon.

If surgery is under consideration, the surgeon will want to carry out extensive preoperative studies and evaluate all the patient's previous history and previous electroencephalographic studies and the laboratory data. If surgery is decided upon, he will try to expose the epileptic focus, delineate it as sharply as possible electroencephalographically, with records made directly from the surface and from the depth of the brain. If the area from which seizure discharges are arising is one in which a structural lesion is present, so much the better. However, in many cases, highly active epileptic processes are structurally invisible and can only be seen electroencephalographically. The therapeutic results obtained by neurosurgeons in the treatment of epilepsy depend upon their skill and judgment in the selection of cases. The extent of the excision and the benefit to be derived from a radical and complete excision must be balanced against the risk of serious deficits. Recordings made immediately post-operatively often show seizure activity that was not present before, but this usually subsides, and it is not necessarily a bad prognostic sign. Sometimes the first postoperative year is a stormy one. Immediately after removal of an epileptogenic focus, anticonvulsant medication must usually be continued. After a year, it may be reduced, and in some cases, particularly when the electroencephalogram no longer shows seizure activity, medication can be discontinued.[5]

Chapter XXVIII

MANAGEMENT OF STATUS EPILEPTICUS

Status epilepticus is a condition in which one seizure follows another in rapid succession without recovery of consciousness between the seizures. The series of convulsions and subsequent stupor may last for hours or even days. Rarely a status is the first sign that a patient has epilepsy. Most usually it occurs as an overwhelming storm of disorder in a patient with seizures which have been more or less satisfactorily controlled with antiepileptic drugs. It constitutes a major medical emergency. The patient should be hospitalized and, if possible, treated in an intensive care unit.

In times past, status was more common than it is today. Better antiepileptic drugs have not only reduced the likelihood of status, but have reduced the mortality from a former high of 50 percent to 11 percent.

Intravenous Dilantin can be tried as a first measure in the effort to end a status, and Nembutal can be tried cautiously. If large amounts of barbiturates are used to suppress the seizures, they may recur hours or even days later, when the barbiturates wear off. Oversedation, particularly with barbiturates, may impair vital functions and may complicate the use of paraldehyde or Valium.

Paraldehyde given by rectum, intramuscularly or intravenously yields excellent results in cases of status. In adults, an initial dose of 1 cc paraldehyde in each buttock can be given and repeated if seizures continue. If they are stopped temporarily and if the status then starts again, the paraldehyde dose can be repeated, 1 cc intravenously at thirty-minute intervals.

With the advent of Valium in intravenous form, a new day dawned in the treatment of status epilepticus.[5,159-162] This drug can also be given intramuscularly, though with somewhat less

143

satisfactory results, in single doses of 10 mg each. Whenever possible, the drug should be administered while the patient is being monitored electroencephalographically. Initial dosages range from 2 to 20 mg injected at the rate of 1 cc (5 mg) per minute and repeated if necessary at fifteen-minute to twenty-minute intervals. The dosage must be based on the patient's age and body weight, on the duration and severity of seizures, and on the observed response to therapy.

Lingual obstruction can be a serious complication in status epilepticus. An airway should be available, and a tracheotomy should be performed if necessary. Aspiration of saliva or stomach contents must be combated. Sometimes with prolonged status the body temperature rises as high as 107 degrees. Intravenous salt solution and dextrose may be needed to prevent dehydration and to prevent the violent exertion from resulting in total exhaustion of energy reserves. The danger attendant on a synergistic action of barbiturates with diazepam may result in a critical hypertension or in respiratory depression. Patients who recover from status epilepticus may die a few days later, usually from cardiac complications.

What has been said here about status epilepticus applies almost exclusively to a grand mal status. A status of psychomotor seizures is extremely rare. Petit mal status is fairly rare and does not usually constitute a medical emergency. The seizures, even if continuous for many hours, are not dangerous. They can usually be prevented by having the patient breathe a mixture of 95% oxygen and 5% carbon dioxide. In rare cases, a petit mal status may change into a grand mal status, but there is no reason to expect such an eventuality unless experience has shown that in the case in question this has occurred previously.[5,161]

Chapter XXIX

WHEN CAN ANTIEPILEPTIC MEDICATION BE DISCONTINUED?

If a patient's seizures have been prevented by antiepileptic medication, he is likely to ask after one year or sometimes less if he can stop taking "drugs." The answer depends on several factors. What type of seizure did he have? If mild and of a type that created no hazards and no social stigma, particularly if the seizures were nocturnal and occurred while the patient was in bed, a trial of reduced medication with final elimination might be attempted. The same holds for an infant or young child; in such a case, one or two more seizures are not likely to have serious consequences. However, "one more seizure" in a school child, college student, housewife, or a person in business may have disastrous results on the patient's educational opportunities, life situation, and earning power.

If the electroencephalogram formerly showed seizure activity and has been normal both awake and asleep, this is a good prognostic sign. If it remains normal for a year, this increases the likelihood that seizures will not return when medication is gradually decreased over a period of two or three weeks and is finally discontinued.

In cases where antiepileptic medication has been effective, it can be regarded as a cheap and practical form of insurance against seizures. In cases where the epileptic disorder is electroencephalographically invisible and where seizures have occurred in spite of a normal electroencephalogram, decisions regarding medication must be based entirely on clinical criteria.[71,73,74]

145

Chapter XXX

TREATMENT OF BEHAVIORAL DISORDERS

Hyperactivity and a state of continuous excitement, sometimes with and sometimes without combativeness, are common complications of epilepsy in childhood. They are particularly common in retarded children with seizures, but they occur also in children with normal or supernormal intelligence. Among children with hyperactivity and severe behavior disturbances, mild tranquilizers, such as meprobamate or Valium may be useful, but usually the powerful chemical restraint of some such substance as chlorpromazine is required. There is no doubt that certain cases, which can only be identified by therapeutic test, respond to amphetamine with a paradoxical quieting effect.

There has been much argument pro and con regarding usefulness of the drug Deaner® in children with behavior disturbances. There is no doubt, however, that in some cases this drug is effective, and it should be tried if behavior disorders are present that cannot be controlled with other medication.

Just as some children show a paradoxical quieting effect with amphetamine, many children, particularly those with brain damage, show paradoxical excitement and irritability when treated with phenobarbital. If a child is hyperactive and is receiving phenobarbital, the gradual reduction of phenobarbital dosage might be tried in order to see whether the hyperactivity decreases, and if so, an attempt might be made to substitute other antiepileptic medications for the phenobarbital.

Adults and, more rarely, children with anterior temporal lobe (psychomotor) epilepsy may have personality disorders or psychiatric symptoms. Such patients may be obsessive, compulsive (sticky), hostile, belligerent, paranoid, or depressed. Indi-

146

cations for the use of tranquilizers in patients with seizures and psychiatric symptoms are essentially the same as for patients with these sypmtoms but without seizures. The attempts to obtain control of seizures with an antiepileptic substance should not be postponed until psychiatric symptoms are reduced. Behavior disturbances and personality disorders in epileptics constitute a separate and distinct therapeutic problem from the seizures. In some cases when seizures are controlled with antiepileptic drugs, the patient's behavior and mental state becomes worse. If the psychiatric symptoms are nonictal, i.e. if they are more or less continuous and do not come in the form of an attack and, particularly, if they are associated with agitation or excitement, rather than depression, there is a fair chance that they will respond to one or more of the tranquilizers. By using both anticonvulsant medication and tranquilizers in combination, the phyiscian may be able to control both sets of symptoms. With the possible exception of Serpasil, the tranquilizers do not subtract significantly from the therapeutic effect of standard antiepileptic drugs. However, they may add to the somnifacient effect of phenobarbital, Mysoline, Mesantoin, the "diones," and the succinamides; therefore the dosage of these may have to be reduced when tranquilizers are prescribed.

Chapter XXXI

PSYCHIATRIC TREATMENT

Erroneous beliefs about the psychological causation of epilepsy and associated personality disorders are so widely held by parents, teachers, social workers, and physicians that many cases of epilepsy are inadequately treated by amateur and professional psychiatrists with major emphasis on psychotherapy and little attention to medication.

Basic misconceptions occasion much unnecessary suffering among parents, for they blame themselves for having said or done something which resulted in their child developing epilepsy. They even call it "causing" the child to have epilepsy. The tragedy is compounded when the patient is made to believe that he can stop his seizures, his rage attacks, his confusional spells, or even his personality disturbances if he only changes his attitudes, rechannels his emotions, or improves his interpersonal relations.

As noted in the foregoing chapters, epilepsy is a medical disorder like diabetes or tuberculosis, and the informed physician cannot subscribe to the prevalent delusion that it has a psychosomatic, psychological, or social basis. Of course, the patient should be dealt with kindly and with consideration, reassured, supported psychologically, and accorded all the rights and privileges of a human being. The nature of his illness should be explained, and he should be helped to understand and accept the part of his trouble that cannot be eliminated.

The major personality disorders and the severe behavior disturbances that occur in some cases of epilepsy are commonly assumed to be caused by feelings of insecurity, by the overprotecting or rejecting attitudes of parents, or by interpersonal reactions of some type. This assumption may be correct in cer-

148

tain cases, but such an interpretation does not take into account the fact that serious personality disorders and severe behavior disturbances occur chiefly in special types and classes of epileptics, particularly in those who have anterior temporal lobe epilepsy or in those who have a type of seizure discharge that indicates a thalamic or hypothalamic origin. The patient's emotional reactions to his seizures, to his family, and to his social situation are less important determinants of psychiatric disorder than the site and the type of the epileptic discharge.

As explained in Chapter XII, continuous psychiatric disorder in patients with psychomotor epilepsy is often a more serious handicap than the patient's seizures. The seizures can, in some cases, be prevented only at the expense of an increase in psychiatric disorder. When personality disturbances or psychosis are a major complication, the patient should be treated with whatever therapy is recommended by an informed psychiatrist. As stated in the preceding chapter, tranquilizers are definitely useful in the treatment of hyperactive, excited, and psychotic epileptics. In some cases of epilepsy-with-psychosis, electroshock, insulin shock, or frontal lobotomy are indicated.

Large islands of ignorance and misunderstanding about epilepsy remain, but there is no doubt that in recent years improvement in the attitudes of the general public, of teachers and administrators, of religious groups, and of employers have improved greatly. This has made the psychological, social, and economic rehabilitation of the epileptic easier and has simplified the task of the psychiatrist who can now encourage an epileptic patient to "come out of his shell," knowing that he is not as likely as formerly to be rebuffed and rejected.

Chapter XXXII

COUNSELLING

What To Do If the Patient Has a Seizure

If an individual has a seizure, the family or other onlookers should understand that there is no need to become panicky, to call the fire department, to call an ambulance to rush the patient into a hospital, or even to send out an immediate emergency call for the doctor. Both the patient and his family should be encouraged to accept the seizure as a manifestation of a type of disorder of brain function which is not in itself dangerous to life. Whether at home, at school, at work, in church, at play, or anywhere, first aid measures should be carried out. Again, one must emphasize that the onlooker should not panic. If it is a child who has the seizure, he can be lifted up carefully and carried to a quiet place, but if the patient is an adult, he should be permitted to have his seizure wherever it occurs. As noted in the First Aid for An Epileptic Seizure, no mouth gag should be used. There is too much danger of broken teeth, pushing the tongue deep into the mouth, or even injury to the fingers of the good samaritan. The head of the patient should be turned so that saliva can run out of his mouth. The patient should be protected from hurting himself by striking a hard object or by burning himself on a hot stove or hot radiator. The onlooker may be able to help the patient as he slides to the ground. However, none of the patient's movements should be completely restrained because the muscular contractions are often so strong that rigid restriction may result in a fracture. Physical force should be kept to a minimum because the patient is likely to react with increased violence if he finds himself tightly restrained. After the seizure, the patient should be left in a quiet place to recover from the postseizure stupor

150

and somnolence. In case the patient is a child, his family should be called. If he is an adult, when he has sufficiently recovered and his state of confusion has cleared, he should be allowed to go on his way, or he should be helped in whatever manner he requests.[189]

FIRST AID FOR AN EPILEPTIC SEIZURE

1. KEEP CALM. The patient is not in pain, is not suffering, and is not in danger.
2. DO NOT be frightened if near an individual with seizures for they are "not catching."
3. DO NOT attempt to stop the attack once it is started. DO NOT try to revive the patient, but let the seizure run its course, which usually takes a few minutes.
4. EASE the person to the floor, loosen tight clothing, but DO NOT restrain his movements.
5. TURN the patient's face to the side to permit release of saliva and make certain that his breathing is not obstructed. A coat may be placed under the head.
6. DO NOT force open the clenched jaws. DO NOT force anything between the patient's teeth. NEVER place a finger in the mouth.
7. DO NOT give the individual anything to drink.
8. STAY with the person until all movement has ceased and stand by until he has recovered consciousness fully and is no longer confused. A small child can be carried to a rest-room, and a larger patient may be allowed to lie until able to talk. If he is tired, permit him to rest, and when he feels better, encourage him to go about his regular activities.
9. DO NOT be frightened if the person with a seizure may appear not to be breathing for a while or breathing poorly.
10. CAREFULLY OBSERVE the details of the attack so this can be reported subsequently to the person's family or to his doctor.
11. If the person is a child, notify the parents. If no one is available, you may call proper authorities. If the attack is an initial one, you may call the doctor.[189]

Diet and General Regime

Other than in exceptional cases (see Ketogenic Diet), the diet of a person with seizures should not be restricted; he can eat a normal diet. Alcohol and tobacco in moderation in most cases do not precipitate seizures nor complicate therapy. No special prescriptions are required for sexual activity. A reasonable balanced amount of sleep, work, and play is as good for the epileptic as it is for anyone. Certainly, one should caution against excessive fatigue, which is a very common cause for precipitative seizures. A rigid schedule is unnecessary for it serves no useful purpose and can only add to the patient's handicap.

As full and active a life as possible should be permitted to the epileptic even when he is on trial medications or when there are changes in medication. Fatigue has already been mentioned as a prominent precipitator of seizures, but extra rest seems to have no true therapeutic value. A busy and interesting schedule usually reduces the number of seizures.

School, Job, Car Driving, and Recreation

The physician's primary effort should be directed toward stopping the seizures. He must not be diverted from this by stepping out of his role as physician in order to act as educational expert, job counselor, or safety engineer. Certainly a child under proper medical care and whose seizures are under good control should not be denied the opportunity to attend school. One cannot guarantee that he will not have a seizure while in school because he spends a large part of his day there, but the teacher should be instructed regarding the nature of her pupil's problem and encouraged to assist him to continue with his education. The teacher can perform an important service by conveying this information to other children in the school, to other teachers, and in some cases, to parents. She should learn also the first aid aspects of the management of the seizure.

An epileptic can do anything that is completely safe for a normal person to do. When his seizures are under good control, it is possible for him to receive a driver's license in every state in the United States. He must be seen at regular intervals by his physician if this privilege is to be continued, and the physician must sign a slip reporting on the patient's condition, which is mailed to the commissioner of motor vehicles, the secretary of state, or some other designated authority. However, if seizures continue or suddenly recur, this driving privilege must be revoked. It is the experience of all who have studied the question, that epileptics whose seizures are properly controlled have fewer automobile accidents than persons without seizures.

Athletic activities should be encouraged, and even body contact sports should not be denied a boy with seizures if he wishes to engage in them. However, boxing is unnecessarily rough. Swimming is to be encouraged, but it should be done where a lifeguard is present; otherwise, institution of a "buddy system" is advisable with all the participants trained in the elements of lifesaving.

Marriage and Heredity

Marriage is a normal goal of adult life, and the physician who is consulted regarding marriage by an epileptic patient usually finds that there is no medical reason or cause for him or her not to marry. However, for a small percentage of epileptics with severe retardation, physical, mental, or both, or with severe, frequent, and uncontrollable seizures, marriage should be discouraged.

With the present effectiveness of contraceptives, the question of marriage and inheritability of epilepsy can be considered separately. There is, in general, a significant hereditary factor in epilepsy. In recent time, it has been "swept under the rug." Lennox pointed out that, in general, the chances are only one in four that an individual with epilepsy will have an epileptic child. This is at least five or ten times as great as the risk run by an nonepileptic. Advice, which is specifically applicable to their case, should be given the prospective marriage couple. Of great importance is the incidence of epilepsy in the marriage partners and in their families and the type or types of epilepsy that are present. (See Fig. 8.) If an epileptic marries another person with a similar problem, the chances of their offspring being affected with epilepsy are doubled. On the other hand, if one prospective marriage partner is completely free of seizures, has no family history of seizures, and has an entirely normal electroencephalogram, the chances of transmitting epilepsy to the offspring are reduced. The marriage partner must always be informed if some type of seizure disorder is present because discovery of the fact after the marriage may produce irrevocable damage to the union.

The presence or absence of epilepsy is not the only factor to be considered when the question of whether an epileptic should or should not have children is at issue. Weight should be given to all the biological assets and liabilities of the patient, the marriage partner, and the families of both.

Employment

Obviously, the employability of an epileptic depends upon his skills and his ability and the degree to which his seizures are controlled, as well as on the type of seizure, whether he has a warning, and whether the seizures are diurnal or nocturnal. However, some employers (fortunately a diminishing number) have a fixed rule against hiring anyone who has had epileptic seizures, even febrile convulsions in infancy. This does not provide the protection that these employers desire because, human nature being what it is, epileptics who think they can get away with it will in many cases deny that they have seizures or that they have ever had seizures. Since most jobs are less hazardous than automobile driving, most enlightened employers have taken the attitude of the authorities dealing with the licensing of persons driving motor vehicles and do employ epileptics who are certified as employable by the treating physicians.

The safety records of large numbers of such patients have been carefully studied, and it has been shown that they have a lower accident rate than nonepileptics employed in comparable work. Of course, hazardous work is contraindicated for persons with uncontrolled seizures, but with proper ingenuity and proper safety precautions, some jobs which might seem to be extremely hazardous can be made safe. For example, a professional steeplejack, who began having seizures in middle life which were fairly well controlled with anticonvulsant medication, was able to continue to work because his two sons, who worked with him, always saw that he was safely strapped into his bosun's chair in such a way that he could not possibly fall out even during a convulsive seizure. Over a period of years, he had several seizures while high in the air without hurting himself. The one serious injury that he received occurred when he had a seizure in his bathroom. Similarly, the employer of a very efficient woman who was a high-speed lathe operator kept her safely at work, in spite of continuing seizures, by providing special safety-engineered guard rails, a screen, and shut-off devices for her lathe.

Personality disorders and paranoid tendencies, sometimes with persistent or episodic outspoken hostility, are often more serious bars to employment in patients with epilepsy than their seizures. Unfortunately, once an employer has had a bad experience with an epileptic who has associated psychiatric symptoms, he is likely to look with disfavor on the employment of all other epileptics. It is also true that, while a very high percentage of epileptics are employable, a small percentage of those who obviously are not give a biased report of the hardships and cruelties to which they have been subjected by fellow employees, foremen, and employers. An informed person usually has no difficulty distinguishing between the facts and the misinterpretation.

Insurance

Unfortunately, the average individual who has seizures is still considered a substandard risk, requiring him then to pay higher premiums than the normal individuals. In life insurance

156 *Epilepsy Handbook*

and individual health and accident insurance coverage, each patient with epilepsy is considered on his own merits. This does not exist in the group insurance plans because when there is blanket accident and health coverage, there is just no specific problem. However, more and more insurance companies are beginning to decrease the requirements for patients who have seizures.

Immigration

Sweeping changes in the Nationality Act, which became law on July 1, 1968, provides that the word "epilepsy" be removed or deleted so that an individual with seizures is no longer refused entry into the United States if he has no other disabling disorder and meets the requirements demanded of all other immigrants.[190,191]

Chapter XXXIII

COMMUNITY ASPECTS OF EPILEPSY

Since epilepsy is a chronic and common disorder, the community must of necessity make some sort of adjustment to it. In ancient times, primitive, unreasoning fear led to the rejection of epileptics. They were considered to be "possessed" (by the devil) and were treated little better than lepers. Later with the development of a greater concern for suffering, but without much increase in understanding, homes or institutions were built to house them. With the dawn of modern medical science, improved understanding and improved treatment made it obvious that the majority of epileptics did not need to be shut up in an institution and were happier living outside in the community. Not only was the noncustodial care of epileptics truly better for epileptics, but it was also demonstrably cheaper and better for the community. The community adjusted with new attitudes; the transition has been a rapid one and is far from complete. As might be expected, parts of the community are more enlightened than others in their attitude towards epileptics, and there are great differences also in the degree of enlightenment from one country to another. Much progress has been achieved through the heroic efforts of lay organizations working for the welfare of epileptics. More about this subject is included in the last paragraph.

From the standpoint of the individual patient, the public's reaction to his illness is crucial. If the patient is a child, he will encounter reactions in school and in his neighborhood and even at home. As an adult, he will be made aware of public attitudes in his social life and in his business contact. If he encounters unkindness and unreasonable discrimination, he is likely to be embittered.[192]

157

Even though it is true that the development of more precise diagnostic procedures and more effective antiepileptic therapy drugs has improved the prospect for most epileptics, there is no doubt that the neglected or rejected child or adult epileptic is likely to develop severe emotional handicaps. Medical management alone is not enough. Prejudicial social attitudes in the community remain to be overcome if a person with seizures is to live, play, and work in a normal environment and to grow up without an impaired image of himself and a hostile attitude toward others. Good medical management, satisfactory vocational guidance, and an enlightened public opinion all work together to provide the maximum success and happiness for a child or adult with seizures.

Once the diagnosis of the patient with epilepsy has been made, the following community resources can be mobilized to lend assistance:

1. Diagnostic evaluation with periodic reevaluation.
2. Medical management and health supervision.
3. Education on a regular or a special basis.
4. Vocational services, which include testing, counseling, job training, and placement.
5. Social work, mental health guidance, and parent counseling.
6. Hospitalization and institutional care.
7. Recreational projects and facilities.

Patient Attitudes

The patient's own attitude must be evaluated carefully, and he must be advised, in terms that he can understand, what to think about his seizures. He must be told what his family, friends, teachers, and employers should know, not about epilepsy in general, but about his seizures in particular. Those with seizures who are unable to accept themselves as worthy individuals need to be concentrated upon especially by social agencies for the purpose of removing, if possible, or at least modifying such detrimental thinking. As stated before, public attitude toward the patient who is an epileptic must be changed in many communities and states, and it is just as important for a physician or a rehabilitation counselor to spend time educating the public as it is to see patients in his office or in the clinic.[193]

Community Programs

An epileptic program is usually started by a group of business-men or community leaders who have seizures or who have someone within their family so affected. Health departments in counties, cities, and states are of great help in disseminating specific information about seizures. With the new impetus in the matter of thorough diagnosis through better examination and more refined management, there is now more and more diminution in the incidence of the emotional presentation. Ideally, no one with seizures should be denied an education, the right to marry, to have children, to drive a car, or to hold public office. Certainly, one should not single out an individual with epilepsy as being different. Therefore, considerable public education is necessary in order that the individual with seizures be accepted with the same composure accorded to those afflicted with tuberculosis, heart trouble, diabetes, or even infantile paralysis.

As Dr. William G. Lennox stated, "Behind the mechanism of seizure lie the subtle attributes and the vicissitudes of each individual epileptic. To clarify the remaining mysteries about seizures and to succour persons subject to them is a long-standing obligation that must be redeemed by physicians, brain scientists, or by men and women of good will."

These men and women of good will certainly exist in every one of our communities, and they are ready to play the essential role in home, office, school, factory, camps, clubs, church, and lay organizations elsewhere. They can be mobilized at any time to assume this obligation, but their task must be directed, and their effort must continue for years if it is to be successful.[194,195]

BIBLIOGRAPHY

1. Bridge, E.M.: *Epilepsy and Convulsive Disorders in Children.* New York, McGraw-Hill, 1949.
2. Livingston, S.: *The Diagnosis and Treatment of Convulsive Disorders in Children.* Springfield, Thomas, 1954.
3. Lennox, W.G.: *Epilepsy and Related Disorders.* Boston, Little, Brown & Co., 1960.
4. Boshes, L.D.: *Early Signs of Neurological Illness,* Consultant. vol. 8, pp. 34–38, 1966.
5. Boshes, L.D., Cohen, M.M., Gibbs, F.A., Grossman, H.J., Klawans, H.L., Metrick, S., and Sugar, O.: The convulsive state, (a symposium). *Curr Med Dig,* 37:35–83, 1970.
6. Janz, D.: *Die Epilepsien.* Stuttgart, Thieme, 1969.
7. Schmidt, R.P., and Wilder, B.J.: *Epilepsy.* Philadelphia, Davis, 1968.
8. Gibbs, F.A., and Gibbs, E.L.: *Atlas of Electroencephalography.* Reading, Addison-Wesley, 1951, vol. I.
9. Gibbs, F.A., and Gibbs, E.L.: *Atlas of Electroencephalography.* Reading, Addison-Wesley, 1952, vol. II.
10. Gibbs, F.A., and Gibbs, E.L.: *Atlas of Electroencephalography.* Reading, Addison-Wesley, 1964, vol. III.
11. Gibbs, F.A., and Gibbs, E.L.: *Medical Electroencephalography.* Reading, Addison-Wesley, 1967.
12. Berger, H.: *Das Elektrenkephalogramm des Menschen.* Nova Acta Leopoldina, 1938, pp. 173–309, vol. 6.
13. Gloor, P., and Berger, H.: On the electroencephalogram of man. *Electroenceph Clin Neurophysiol,* Suppl 28, Amsterdam, Elsevier, 1969.
14. Jackson, J.H.: Epilepsy and epileptiform convulsions. In Taylor, J. (Ed.): *Selected Writings.* London, Hodder and Stoughton, 1931, vol. I.
15. Gibbs, F.A., Gibbs, E.L., and Lennox, W.G.: Epilepsy: A paroxysmal cerebral dysrhythmia. *Brain,* 60:377–388, 1937.
16. Gibbs, F.A., and Gibbs, E.L.: Age factor in epilepsy: A summary and synthesis. *New Eng J Med,* 269:1230–1236, 1963.
17. Toman, J.E.P., and Boshes, L.D.: Normal and pathological changes in the electroencephalogram of older patients. *Sci Int,* 2:4, 1954.
18. Boshes, L.D.: Epilepsy in the 7th decade. *JAMA,* 189:72, 1964.
19. Moore, F.J., Kellaway, P., Kagawa, N.: Metrazol activation as a

diagnostic adjunct in electroencephalography, a re-evaluation. *Neurology, 4:*325–338, 1954.

20. Ulett, G.A., Johnson, L.C., and Mills, W.B.: Pattern stability and relationship among electroencephalographic "activation" techniques. *Electroenceph Clin Neurophysiol, 11:*251–266, 1959.

21. Brandt, H., Brandt, S., and Vollmond, K.: EEG response to photic stimulation in 120 normal children. *Epilepsia, 2:*313–317, 1961.

22. Wacaser, L.: Photic activation of the electroencephalogram. *Clin Electroenceph, 1:*32–35, 1970.

23. Boshes, L.D.: Inflammatory and infectious diseases of the nervous system. *Tice—Practice of Medicine vol. X Chapt XIX pp.* 1–56, 1970.

24. Boshes, L.D.: A review of fungus infections of the central nervous system. *Mycopathologia, 3:*215–237, 1960.

25. Boshes, L.D.: Sarcoidosis of the nervous system. *Dis Nerv Syst, 23:*683–687, 1962.

26. Boshes, L.D., Sherman, I.C., Hesser, C.J., Milzer, A., and McClain, H.: Fungus infections of the central nervous system, experience in treatment of cryptococcosis and cycloheximide (actidione.) *Arch Neurol Psychiat, 75:*175–190, 1956.

27. Boshes, L.D., Sherman, I.C., Hesser, C.J., Milzer, A., and McClain, H.: Alterations in the central nervous system with various fungus infections. *Trans Amer Neurol Ass, 80:*178, 1955.

28. Gibbs, E.L., Fleming, M.M., and Gibbs, F.A.: Diagnosis and prognosis of hypsarhythmia and infantile spasms. *Pediatrics, 13:*66–73, 1954.

29. Livingston, S., Bridge, E.M., and Kajdi, L.: Febrile convulsions: A clinical study with special reference to heredity and prognosis. *J Pediat, 31:*509–512, 1947.

30. Garvin, J.S.: Significance of convulsions with fever. *Clin Electroenceph, 1:*41–44, 1970.

31. Gibbs, F.A., Gibbs, E.L., and Lennox, W.G.: The influence of the blood sugar level on the wave and spike formation of petit mal epilepsy. *Arch Neurol Psychiat, 41:*1111–1116, 1939.

32. Lennox, W.G., and Davis, J.P.: Clinical correlates of the fast and the slow spike-wave electroencephalogram. *Pediat, 5:*626–644, 1950.

33. Penfield, W., and Jasper, H.: *Epilepsy and the Functional Anatomy of the Human Brain.* Boston, Little, Brown and Co., 1954.

34. Bennett, F.E.: Intracarotid and intravertebral Metrazol in petit mal epilepsy. *Neurol, 3:*668–673, 1953.

35. Williams, D.: The thalamus and epilepsy. *Brain, 88:*539–556, 1965.

36. Gloor, P.: Generalized cortico-reticular epilepsies: Some considera-

tions on the pathophysiology of generalized bilaterally synchronous spike and wave discharges. *Epilepsia, 9:*249–263, 1968.

37. Gibbs, F.A., Davis, H., and Lennox, W.G., The electro-encephalogram in epilepsy and conditions of impaired consciousness. *Arch Neurol Psychiat, 34:*1133–1148, 1935.

38. Bickford, R.G., and Klass, D.W.: Sensory precipitation and reflex epilepsy. In Jasper, Ward, and Pope (Eds.): *Basic Mechanisms of Epilepsy.* Boston, Little, Brown and Co., 1969, pp. 543–573.

39. Metrakos, K., and Metrakos, J.D.: Is the centrencephalic E.E.G. inherited as a dominant? *Electroenceph Clin Neurophysiol, 13:*289, 1961.

40. Metrakos, K., and Metrakos, J.D.: Genetics of convulsive disorders, II, Genetic and electroencephalographic studies in centrencephalic epilepsy. *Neurol, 11:*474–483, 1961.

41. Gibbs, E.L., and Gibbs, F.A.: Electroencephalographic evidence of thalamic and hypothalamic epilepsy. *Neurol, 1:*136–144, 1951.

42. Kooi, K.A.: Involuntary movements associated with fourteen and six per second positive waves: Report of a case with electroencephalographic studies. *Neurol, 18:*997–1002, 1968.

43. Holbrook, T.J.: A case with 6 per second positive spike discharges and temporally associated clinical manifestations. *Clin Electroenceph, 1:*36–40, 1970.

44. Hughes, J.R.: In Wilson, W.P. (Ed.): *A Review of the Positive Spike Phenomenon in Applications of Electroencephalography to Psychiatry.* Durham, Duke University Press, 1965, pp. 54–101.

45. Gibbs, F.A., and Gibbs, E.L.: Fourteen and six per second positive spikes. *Electroenceph Clin Neurophysiol, 15:*553–558, 1963.

46. Metcalf, D.R.: Controlled studies of the incidence and significance of 14 and 6 per second positive spiking. *Electroenceph Clin Neurophysiol, 15:*160–163, 1963.

47. Gibbs, F.A.: The electroencephalogram in mental retardation. In Carter, C.H. (Ed.): *Medical Aspects of Mental Retardation.* Springfield, Thomas, 1965.

48. Schwade, E.D., and Geiger, S.G.: Matricide with electroencephalographic evidence of thalamic or hypothalamic disorder. *Dis Nerv Syst, 14:*18–20, 1953.

49. Winfield, D.L., and Ozturk, O.: Electroencephalographic findings in matricide (a case report). *Dis Nerv Syst, 20:*176–178, 1959.

50. Thomas, J.: A rare electroencephalographic pattern: The six per second spike and wave discharge. *Neurol, 7:*438–442, 1957.

51. Hughes, J.R., Schlagenhauf, R.E., and Magos, M.: Electro-clinical correlations in the six per second spike-and-wave complex. *Electroenceph Clin Neurophysiol, 18:*71–77, 1965.

52. Hill, J.N.D., and Parr, G.: *Electroencephalography*, London, Macdonald, 1963.
53. Gibbs, F.A., Rich, C.L., and Gibbs, E.L.: Psychomotor variant type of seizure discharge. *Neurol, 13*:991–998, 1963.
54. Garvin, J.S.: Psychomotor variant pattern. *Dis Nerv Syst, 29*:307–309, 1968.
55. Lombroso, C.T., *et al.*: Steroids in healthy youths: Controlled study of 14 and six per second positive spiking. *Neurol, 16*:1152–1158, 1966.
56. Schwartz, I.H., and Lombroso, C.T.: 14 and 6 per second positive spiking (steroids) in the electroencephalograms of primary school pupils. *J Pediat, 72*:678–682, 1968.
57. Walter, R.D., *et al.*: A controlled study of the 14 and 6 per second EEG pattern. *Arch Gen Psychiat, 2*:559–566, 1960.
58. Thomas, J.E., and Klass, D.W.: Six per second spike-and-wave pattern in the electroencephalogram: A reappraisal of its clinical significance. *Neurol, 18*:587–593, 1968.
59. Gibbs, F.A.: Unpublished study.
60. Glenn, C.G., Knuth, R., and Virgil, M., Sr.: Electroencephalographic findings in children with juvenile duodenal ulcer. *Dis Nerv Syst, 27*:662–664, 1966.
61. Reilly, E.L., *et al.*: Some observations on the EEG in allergic children. *Southern Med J, 61*:880, 1968.
62. Winfield, D.L., and Aivazian, G.H.: EEG changes associated with pseudohypertrophic muscular dystrophy. *Southern Med J, 51*: 1251–1259, 1958.
63. Perlstein, M.A., *et al.*: Electroencephalogram and myopathy. Relation between muscular dystrophy and related diseases. *JAMA, 173*: 1329–1333, 1960.
64. Gibbs, E.L., Gibbs, F.A., and Hirsch, W.: Rarity of 14 and 6 per second positive spiking among mongoloids. *Neurol, 14*:581–583, 1964.
65. Rodin, E.A.: Familial occurrence of 14 and 6 per second positive spike phenomenon. *Electroenceph Clin Neurophysiol, 17*:566–570, 1964.
66. Fois, A., Borgheresi, S., and Luti, E.: Possibilita di un sub-strato familiare nella patogenesi degli attacchi neurovegetativi. *Riv Clin Pediat, 79*:72–82, 1967.
67. Petersen, I., and Akesson, H.O.: EEG studies on siblings of children showing 14 and 6 per second positive spikes. *Acta Genet (Basel), 18*:163–169, 1968.
68. Penfield, W., and Erickson, T.C.: *Epilepsy and Cerebral Localization.* Springfield, Thomas, 1941.
69. Fois, A., and Lippi, A.: Nonictal symptoms associated with severe

electroencephalographic epileptiform abnormalities. *Clin Electro-enceph*, 1:22–31, 1970.

70. Gibbs, F.A., et al.: Relation between specific types of occipital dysrhythmia and visual defects. *Johns Hopkins Med J*, 122:343–349, 1968.

71. Gibbs, F.A., and Gibbs, E.L.: Clinical correlates and prognostic significance of various types of mid-temporal focus. *Clin Electroenceph*, 1:45–64, 1970.

72. Ursin, H.: The temporal lobe substrate of fear and anger. A review of recent stimulation and ablation studies in animals and humans. *Acta Psychiat, Scand*, 35:378–396, 1960.

73. Gibbs, F.A., et al.: Electroencephalographic and clinical aspects of cerebral palsy. *Pediatrics*, 32:73–84, 1963.

74. Gibbs, E.L., Gillen, H.W., and Gibbs, F.A.: Disappearance and migration of epileptic foci in childhood. *Amer J Dis Child*, 88: 596–603, 1954.

75. Gibbs, E.L., Gibbs, F.A., and Fuster, B.: Psychomotor epilepsy. *Arch Neurol Psychiat*, 60:331–339, 1948.

76. Belinson, L., and Cowie, W.S.: Electroencephalographic characteristics of institutionalized epileptics. *Amer J Ment Defic*, 52:9–15, 1947.

77. Earl, K.M., Baldwin, M., and Penfield, W.: Incisural sclerosis and temporal lobe seizures produced by hippocampal herniation at birth. *Arch Neurol Psychiat*, 69:27–42, 1953.

78. Green, J.R., Duisberg, R.E.H., and McGrath, W.B.: Focal epilepsy of psychomotor type. A preliminary report of observations on effects of surgical therapy. *J Neurosurg*, 8:157–172, 1951.

79. Scoville, W.B., et al.: Observations on medial temporal lobectomy and uncotomy in the treatment of psychotic states. Preliminary review of 19 operative cases compared with 60 frontal lobotomy and undercutting cases. *Res Publ Ass Nerv Ment Dis*, 31:347–369, 1953.

80. Terzian, H.: Observations on the clinical symptomoatology of bilateral partial or total removal of the temporal lobes in man. In Baldwin, M., and Bailey, P.: *Temporal Lobe Epilepsy*. Springfield, Thomas, 1958, pp. 510–529.

81. Gibbs, F.A., Amador, L., and Rich, C.: In Baldwin, M., and Bailey, P.: *Temporal Lobe Epilepsy*. Springfield, Thomas, 1958, pp. 358–367.

82. Green, J.R., and Sheets, D.G.: Surgery of epileptogenic lesions of the temporal lobe. *Arch Neurol (Chicago)*, 10:135–148, 1964.

83. Falconer, M.A.: The surgical treatment of temporal lobe epilepsy. *Neurochirurgia (Stuttgart)*, 8:161–172, 1965.

84. Forster, F.M.: Conditioning of cerebral dysrhythmia induced by pattern presentation and eye closure. *Cond Ref*, 2:236, 1967.

85. Stevens, H., and Shorey, M.: Masked epilepsy. *Clin Proc Child Hosp,* 21:315–323, 1965.

86. Alvarez, W.C.: *Practical Leads to Puzzling Diagnosis.* Philadelphia, Lippincott, 1958.

87. Low, N.L., Gibbs, E.L., and Gibbs, F.A.: Electroencephalographic findings in breath-holding spells. *Pediatrics,* 15:595–599, 1955.

88. Engel, G.L.: *Fainting: Physiological and Psychological Considerations,* 2nd ed. Springfield, Thomas, 1962.

89. Forster, F.M., Roseman, E., and Gibbs, F.A.: Electroencephalogram accompanying hyperactive carotid sinus reflex and orthostatic-syncope. *Arch Neurol Psychiat,* 48:957–967, 1942.

90. Ferris, E.B., Capps, R.B., and Weiss, S.: Carotid sinus syncope and its bearing on the mechanism of the unconscious state and convulsions. *Medicine,* 14:377–456, 1935.

91. Gastaut, H., Vigouroux, R., and Dell, M.: Polygraphic study of carotid sinus hypersensitivity produced by extra sinus stimulation (compression of the carotid sinus). In Gastaut, H., and Meyers, J.S.: *Cerebral Anoxia and the Electroencephalogram.* Springfield, Thomas, 1961, pp. 485–507.

92. Gibbs, F.A., and Murray, E.L.: Hypoglycemic convulsions. *Electroenceph Clin Neurophysiol,* 6:674–678, 1954.

93. Etheridge, J.E., and Millichap, J.G.: Hypoglycemia and seizures in childhood. Etiologic significance of primary cerebral lesions. *Neurol,* 14:397–404, 1964.

94. Troy, J.M.: Hypsarhythmia accompanying tetany of the newborn. *J Indiana Med Ass,* 62:1216–1217, 1969.

95. Apter, N.S., et al.: Alterations of cerebral functions in pheochromocytoma. *Neurol,* 1:283–292, 1951.

96. Wikler, A., et al.: Electroencephalographic changes associated with chronic alcoholic intoxication and the alcoholic abstinence syndrome. *Amer J Psychol,* 113:106–114, 1956.

97. Greenblatt, M., Levin, S., and Cori, F. di: The electroencephalogram associated with chronic alcoholism, alcoholic psychosis and alcoholic convulsions. *Arch Neurol Psychiat,* 52:290–295, 1944.

98. Wikler, A., et al.: Electroencephalograms during cycles of addiction to barbiturates in man. *Electroenceph Clin Neurophysiol,* 7:1–13, 1955.

99. Daly, D.D., and Yoss, R.E.: The treatment of narcolepsy with methyl phenylpiperidylacetate: A preliminary report. *Mayo Clin,* 31:620, 1956.

100. Kravitz, H., et al.: A study of head-banging in infants and children. *Dis Nerv Syst,* 21:203–208, 1960.

101. Meduna, von L.: Versuche über die biologieche Beeinflussung des

ablaufes der Schizophrenia. I. Cardiazol-Krampfe. *Z ges Neurol Psychiat, 152:*235–262, 1935.

102. Lennox, W.G.: The heredity of epilepsy as told by relatives and twins. *JAMA, 146:*529–536, 1951.
103. Kimball, O.P.: On the inheritance of epilepsy, *Wisconsin Med J, 53:*271–276, 1954.
104. Bray, P.F., and Wiser, W.C.: Evidence for a genetic etiology of temporal-central abnormalities in focal epilepsy. *New Eng J Med, 271:*926–933, 1964.
105. Walker, A.E.: *Post-traumatic Epilepsy.* Springfield, Thomas, 1949.
106. Radermecker, J. and Poser, C.M.: The significance of repetative paroxysmal electroencephalographic patterns. Their specificity in subacute sclerosing leukoencephalitis. *World Neurol, 1:*422–435, 1960.
107. Gibbs, F.A., and Reid, D.E.: Electroencephalogram in pregnancy. *Amer J Obstet Gynec, 44:*672–675, 1942.
108. Radermecker, J.: Systématique et électroencéphalographie des encéphalites et encéphalopathies. *Electroenceph Clin Neurophysiol,* Suppl. 5, Masson & Cie, Paris, 1956.
109. Gibbs, F. A., et al.: Electroencephalographic abnormality in "uncomplicated" childhood diseases. *JAMA, 171:*1050–1055, 1959.
110. Greenblatt, M., and Levin, S.: Factors affecting the electroencephalogram of patients with neuro-syphilis. *Amer J Psychiat 102:* 40–48, 1945.
111. Penfield, W., and Humphreys, S.: Epileptogenic lesions of the brain. *Arch Neurol Psychiat, 43:*240–261, 1940.
112. Jennett, W.B., and Lewin, W.: Traumatic epilepsy after closed head injuries. *J Neurol Neurosurg Psychiat, 23:*295–301, 1960.
113. Gibbs, F.A., Wegner, W.R., and Gibbs, E.L.: The electroencephalogram in post-traumatic epilepsy. *Amer J Psychiat, 100:*738–749, 1944.
114. Masquin, A., and Courjon, J.: Prognostic factors in post-traumatic epilepsy. *Epilepsia, 4:*285–297, 1963.
115. Chusid, J.G., and De Gutierrez-Mahoney, C.G.: The electroencephalogram in head injuries with subdural hematoma. *Neurol, 6:*11–21, 1956.
116. Gibbs, F.A.: The frequency with which variously located tumors produce certain symptoms. *Arch Neurol Psychiat, 28:*969–989, 1932.
117. Penfield, W., and Erickson, T.C.: *Epilepsy and Cerebral Localization.* Springfield, Thomas, 1941.
118. Guvener, A., Bagchi, B.K., Kooi, K.A., and Calhoun, H.D.: Mental and seizure manifestations in relation to brain tumors, A statistical study. *Epilepsia, 5:*166–176, 1964.
119. Gibbs, E.L., and Gibbs, F.A.: Extreme spindles, correlation of elec-

troencephalographic sleep patterns with mental retardation. *Science, 138:*1106–1107, 1962.

120. Boshes, L.D.: Days of our years. *Illinois Med J, 126:*712–756, 1967.
121. Boshes, L.D.: The medical treatment of epilepsy in children. *Chicago Med, 72:*347–351, 1969.
122. Hauptmann, A.: Luminal bei Epilepsie. *München Med Wschr, 59:* 1907–1909, 1912.
123. Arieff, A.J.: Twelve year resume in a clinic for epilepsy. *Dis Nerv Syst, 12:*19, 1951.
124. Livingston, S., and Pearson, P.H.: Bromides in the treatment of epilepsy in children. *Amer Med Ass J Dis Child, 86:*717, 1953.
125. Merritt, H.H., and Putnam, T.J.: Sodium diphenyl hydantoinate in treatment of convulsive disorders. *JAMA, 111:*1068–1073, 1938.
126. Merritt, H.H., and Carter, S.: Symposium on medical therapeutics: Anticonvulsant drugs. *Med Clin N Amer, 34:*341–350, 1950.
127. Steinberg, A., and Boshes, L.D.: Effect of Dilantin on gingival tissue. Unpublished observations.
128. Morrell, F., Bradley, W., and Ptashne, M.: Effect of drugs on discharge characteristics of chronic epileptogenic lesions. *Neurol, 9:*492–498, 1959.
129. Handley, R., and Stewart, A.S.R.: Mysoline, A new drug in the treatment of epilepsy. *Lancet, 1:*742–744, 1952.
130. Smith, B.H., and McNaughton, F.L.: Mysoline, a new anticonvulsant drug: Its value in refractory cases of epilepsy, *Canad MAJ, 68:*464–468, 1953.
131. Loscalzo, A.E.: Treatment of epileptic patients with a combination of 3 methyl, 5-5 phenyl-ethyl hydantoin and phenobarbital. *J Nerv Ment Dis, 101:*537–544, 1945.
132. Fetterman, J., and Victoroff, V.: Mesantoin in epilepsy: A three year study. *Dis Nerv Syst, 10:*355–359, 1949.
133. Garvin, J.S., and Gibbs, F.A.: Mesantoin toxicity (a clinical note). *Dis Nerv Syst, 11:*48–50, 1950.
134. Butler, T.C.: Quantitative studies of the physiological disposition of 3-methyl-5-ethyl-5 phenyl hydantoin (Mesantoin) and 5-ethyl-5 phenyl hydantoin (Nirvanol). *J Pharmacol Exp Ther, 109:*340–345, 1953.
135. American Medical Association Council on Drugs: *New and Nonofficial Drugs.* Philadelphia, Lippincott, 1963.
136. Lennox, W.G.: The petit mal epilepsies; their treatment with Tridione. *JAMA, 129:*1069–1073, 1945.
137. Perlstein, M.A., and Andelman, M.B.: Tridione, its use in convulsive and related disorders. *J Pediat, 29:*20–40, 1946.
138. Davis, J.P., and Lennox, W.G.: A comparison of Paradione and Tridione in the treatment of epilepsy. *J Pediat, 34:*273–278, 1949.

139. Bloom, W., Lynch, J.P., and Brick, H.: Mesantoin poisoning with aplastic anemia and recovery. *JAMA, 138*:498–499, 1948.
140. Zimmerman, F.T., and Burgemeister, B.B.: Use of N-methyl-a-a-methyl-phenyl succinimide in treatment of psychomotor epilepsy. *Arch Neurol Psychiat, 72*:720–725, 1954.
141. Zimmerman, F.T.: Evaluation of N-Methyl-a-a-methyl-phenyl succinimide in the treatment of petit mal epilepsy. *New York J Med, 56*:1460, 1956.
142. Kiorboe, E., Paludan, J., Trolle, E., and Overad, E.: Zarontin (ethosuximide) in the treatment of petit mal and related disorders. *Epilepsia, 5*:83–89, 1964.
143. Zimmerman, F.T., and Burgemeister, B.B.: A new drug for petit mal epilepsy. *Neurol, 8*:769–775, 1958.
144. Heathfield, K.W.G., and Jewesbury, E.C.O.: Treatment of petit mal with ethosuximide. *Brit Med J, 2*:565, 1961.
145. Millichap, J.G.: Milontin, a new drug in the treatment of petit mal. *Lancet, 2*:907–910, 1952.
146. Zimmerman, F.T.: Use of methylphenyl succinimide in treatment of petit mal epilepsy. *Arch Neurol Psychiat, 56*:156–162, 1951.
147. Gibbs, F.A., Everett, G.M., and Richards, R.K.: Phenurone in epilepsy. *Dis Nerv Syst, 10*:47–49, 1949.
148. Tyler, M.V., and King, E.J.: Phenacemide in treatment of epilepsy. *JAMA, 147*:17–21, 1951.
149. Forster, F.M.: Therapy in psychomotor epilepsy. *JAMA, 145*:211–215, 1951.
150. Livingston, S.: *Drug Therapy for Epilepsy.* Springfield, Thomas, 1966.
151. American Medical Association Council on Drugs: *New and Nonofficial Drugs.* Philadelphia, Lippincott, 1958.
152. Berris, H.: Mebaral as an anticonvulsant. *Neurol, 4*:116–119, 1954.
153. Perlstein, M.A.: Gemonil (5.5-diethyl 1-methyl. barbituric acid). New drug for convulsive and related disorders. *Pediatrics, 5*:448–451, 1950.
154. Perlstein, M.A.: Metharbital (Gemonil) in myoclonic spasms of infancy and related disorders. *Amer Med Ass J Dis Child, 93*:425, 1957.
155. Schwade, E.D., Richards, R.K., and Everett, G.M.: Peganone, a new antiepileptic drug. *Dis Nerv Syst, 17*:155–158, 1956.
156. American Medical Association Council on Drugs: *New and Nonofficial Drugs.* Philadelphia, Lippincott, 1961.
157. Watson, C.W., Bowker, R., and Calish, C.: Effect of chlordiazepoxide on epileptic seizures. *JAMA, 188*:212–216, 1964.
158. Livingston, S., Pauli, L., and Murphy, J.B.: Ineffectiveness of chlordiazepoxide hydrochloride in epilepsy. *JAMA, 177*:243, 1961.
159. Gastaut, H., Naquet, R., Poire, R., and Tassinari, C.A.: Treatment of

status epilepticus with diazepam (Valium). *Epilepsia, 6*:167–182, 1965.

160. Lombroso, C.T.: Treatment of status epilepticus with diazepam, *Neurol, 19*:629–634, 1969.

161. Boshes, L.D.: Treatment of status epilepticus. *Med Trib Med News,* 6:12, 1965.

162. Bell, D.S.: Dangers of treatment of status epilepticus with diazepam. *Brit Med J, 1*:159–161, 1969.

163. Blom, S.: Tic douloureux treated with a new anticonvulsant; experiences with g-32883: *Arch Neurol, 9*:285–290, 1963.

164. Dolessio, D.J.: Medical treatment of tic douloureux. *Neurol, 16*:303, 1966.

165. Hernandez-Peon, R.: Anticonvulsant action of g-32883 CINP Congress Munich. Amsterdam, Elsevier, 1962, pp. 303–311.

166. Kienast, H.W., and Boshes, L.D.: Clinical trials of carbamazepine suppressing pain. *Headache, 8*:1–6, 1968.

167. Gibbs, F.A., and Anderson, E.M.: Treatment of hypsarhythmia and infantile spasms with a Librium analogue. *Neurol, 15*:1173–1176, 1965.

168. Anderson, E.M., Gibbs, F.A., and Boshes, L.D.: Anticonvulsant action of Mogadon, a Librium analogue. *Proc Inst Med Chic, 26*:82, 1966.

169. Millichap, J.G., and Ortiz, W.R.: Nitrazepam in myoclonic epilepsies. *Amer J Dis Child, 112*:242–248, 1968.

170. Peterson, W.G.: Clinical study of Mogadon. *Neurol, 17*:878–913, 1967.

171. King, L.J., Lowry, O.H., Passoneau, J.V., and Venson, V.: Effects of convulsants on energy reserves in the cerebral cortex. *J Neurochem, 14*:599–611, 1967.

172. Wada, T., Sato, T., and Morita, S.: Diamox (acetazolamide) in treatment of epilepsy. *Dis Nerv Syst, 18*:110–117, 1957.

173. Sorel, L., and Dusaucy-Bauloye, A.: A propos de 21 cas d' hypsarhythmia de Gibbs, Traitement spectaculaire par l'ACTH. *Rev Neurol, 99*:136, 1956.

174. Gibbs, F.A. (Ed.): *Molecules and Mental Health.* Philadelphia, Lippincott, 1959.

175. Stamps, F.W., *et al.*: Treatment of hypsarhythmia with ACTH. *JAMA, 171*:408–411, 1959.

176. Miribel, J., and Poirier, F.: Effects of ACTH and adrenocortical hormone in juvenile epilepsy. *Epilepsia, 2*:345–353, 1961.

177. Millichap, J.G., and Bickford, R.G.: Infantile spasms, hypsarhythmia and mental retardation. Response to corticotropin and its relation to age and etiology in 21 patients. *JAMA, 182*:523, 1962.

178. Fois, A. and Lippi, A.: Nonictal symptoms associated with severe elec-

troencephalographic epileptiform abnormalities. *Clin Electroenceph,* 1:22–31, 1970.

179. Anderson, E.M.: Personal communication.
180. Merlis, S.: Diamox: A carbonic anhydrase inhibitor, its use in epilepsy. *Neurology,* 4:863–868, 1954.
181. Millichap, J.G., Woodbury, D.M., and Goodman, L.S.: Mechanism of the anticonvulsant action of acetazolamide, a carbonic anhydrase inhibitor. *J Pharmacol Exp Ther, 115:*251–258, 1955.
182. Gray, W.D., and Rauh, C.E.: The anticonvulsant action of inhibitors of carbonic anhydrase, relation to endogenous amines in brain. *J Pharmacol Exp Ther, 155:*127–134, 1967.
183. Lennox, W.G.: *Science and Seizures.* New York, Harper, 1941.
184. Sibley, W.A., Tucker, H.J., and Randt, C.T.: Quinacrine in the treatment of refractory petit mal epilepsy. *New Eng J Med,* 267:332–336, 1962.
185. Perlstein, M.A.: Use of meprobamate (Miltown) in convulsive and related disorders. *JAMA, 161:*1040–1044, 1956.
186. Peterman, M.G.: Ketogenic diet in the treatment of epilepsy. *Amer J Dis Child,* 28:28–33, 1924.
187. Keith, H.M.: *Convulsive Disorders in Children.* Boston, Little, Brown & Co., 1963.
188. Bailey, P., Green, J.R., Amador, L., and Gibbs, F.A.: Treatment of psychomotor states by anterior temporal lobectomy, a report of progress. Psychiatric treatment. *Assoc Res Nerv Ment Dis Proc, 31:*341–346, 1953.
189. Boshes, L.D.: First aid for an epileptic seizure, (chart), for use in hospitals, schools, factories, playgrounds, etc. Consultation Clinic for Epilepsy, University of Illinois, College of Medicine.
190. Barrow, R.L., and Fabing, H.D.: *Epilepsy and the Law,* 2nd ed. New York, Hoeber Medical Division, Harper, Row & Co., 1966.
191. Boshes, L.D.: Epilepsy and the law. *Dis Nerv Syst,* 26:569–573, 1965.
192. Boshes, L.D.: Community problems, Symposium on Epilepsy. Barrow Neurological Institute publication, 1966, pp. 44–47.
193. Boshes, L.D.: Problems of patient adjustment, Symposium on Epilepsy. Barrow Neurological Institute publication, 1966, pp. 46–47.
194. Boshes, L.D.: Community aspects of epilepsy. *Curr Med Dig,* 32:955–963, 1965.
195. Boshes, L.D., and Kienast, H.W.: Community aspects of epilepsy, a modern approach. *Illinois Med J, 138:*140–147, 1970.

NAME INDEX

Aivazian, G.H., 48
Akesson, H.O., 48, 86
Alvarez, W.C., 63
Amador, L., 59, 141
American Medical Association Council
  on Drugs, 123, 127, 130, 132, 133
Andelman, M.B., 124, 125
Anderson, E.M., 134, 135
Apter, N.S., 73
Arieff, A.J., 118, 139

Bagchi, B.K., 104
Bailey, P., 141
Baldwin, M., 58
Barrow, R.L., 156
Belinson, L., 57
Bell, D.S., 133, 143
Bennett, F.E., 33
Berger, H., 3
Berris, H., 131
Bickford, R.G., 35, 61, 135
Blom, S., 134
Bloom, W., 126
Borgheresi, S., 48, 86
Boshes, L.D., 3, 4, 18, 21, 95, 117, 120,
  133, 134, 142–144, 151, 156, 157,
  158, 159
Bowker, R., 133
Bradley, W., 121
Brandt, H., 18
Brandt, S., 18
Bray, P.F., 86
Brick, H., 126
Bridge, E.M., vii, 25, 103
Burgemeister, B.B., 128
Butler, T.C., 123

Calhoun, H.D., 104
Calish, C., 133
Capps, E.B., 68
Carter, S., 119, 120

Chusid, J.G., 100
Cohen, M.M., 4, 142, 143, 144
di Cori, F., 74
Courjon, J., 98
Cowie, W.S., 57

Daly, D.D., 75
Davis, H., 34
Davis, J.P., 30, 32, 126, 127
De Gutierrez-Mahoney, C.G., 100
Dell, M., 68
Dolessio, D.J., 134
Duisberg, R.E.H., 59
Dusaucy-Bauloye, A., 135

Earl, K.M., 58
Engel, G.L., 67
Erickson, T.C., 50, 103, 104
Etheridge, J.E., 72, 88
Everett, G.M., 129, 130, 132

Fabing, H.D., 156
Falconer, M.A., 59
Ferris, E.B., 68
Fetterman, J., 122
Fleming, M.M., 22
Fois, A., 48, 50, 86, 135
Forster, F.M., 60, 62, 68, 69, 129
Fuster, B., 54

Garvin, J.S., 25, 26, 27, 45, 123
Gastaut, H., 68, 133, 143
Geiger, S.G., 44
Gibbs, E.L., vii, 6, 9, 18, 22, 30, 32, 37,
  40–42, 45, 48, 52, 54, 57, 58, 65, 66,
  70, 75, 89, 93, 94, 97, 103, 104, 107,
  109, 112, 145
Gibbs, F.A., vii, 4, 6, 9, 18, 22, 30, 32,
  34, 37, 40–42, 44, 45, 48, 51, 52, 54,
  57–59, 65, 66, 68–70, 72, 75, 89, 90,
  92–94, 97, 103, 104, 107–109, 112,
  123, 129, 130, 134, 135, 141–145

171

SUBJECT INDEX

A

Abscess
  brain, 95–97
  cutaneous, on face, 126
Absences, *see* Petit mal
Accessory drugs, 133–140
  see also ACTH, Aralen, Atabrine,
    Bromides, Caffeine, Corticosteroids
    Desoxyn, Dexedrine, Diamox, Lib-
    rium, Mellaril, Meprobamate, Mo-
    gadon, Serpasil, Stelazine, Tegre-
    tol, Thorazine, Valium, and Ves-
    prin
Accident rates, 154, 155
Acetazolamide, *see* Diamox
Acidosis, and
  Diamox, 136
  ketogenic diet, 140
Acneform eruption, with
  bromides, 140
  Tridione, 126
ACTH
  accessory drug, 24, 117, 135, 136
  dosage, 135
  hypsarhythmia, 24, 135, 136
  infection, etiology, 113
  normalize EEG, 135
Activation procedures, 18
  see also Photic stimulation
Addiction, phenobarbital, 118, 119
  see also Withdrawal seizures
Adolescents, and
  control subjects, 43
  epilepsy, types, 8, 33, 35, 42, 48, 52
  masked epilepsy, 63
  mental retardation, 108
  see also Age factor
Adults, and
  control subjects, 43
  epilepsy, types, 8, 9, 16, 18, 30, 35,
    45, 51, 54, 57

etiology, 92, 98, 100, 102, 103
masked epilepsy, 63
mental retardation, 108
nonepileptic conditions, 70, 78, 79
personality disorder, 146
therapy, 118–121, 124, 127, 132–
  134, 136, 137, 140, 143, 145
  see also Age factor
Adversive seizures, 52
Age factor, 8, 9
  breath-holding, 66
  cerebral palsy, 110, 111
  febrile convulsions, 25, 26
  focal discharge, 50–52
  fourteen and six, 42
  hypsarhythmia, 23
  mental retardation, 108
  myoclonic seizures, 37
  petit mal, 33, 35
  petit mal variant, 30, 32
  pseudo petit mal, 27
  psychomotor, 57
  six per second spike-and-wave, 45
  surgical treatment, 141
  trauma, 97, 98
Agranulocytosis, 134
Akinetic seizures, 30, 32
  sensory-induced, 61, 62
  treatment, 127, 128, 130
Alcohol and seizures, 73, 74, 152
Allergy, 48, 90, 91
Amblyopia, 51
Amnesia, with
  auras, 65
  grand mal, 15
  psychomotor, 54, 56
  trauma, 96
Amphetamine
  accessory drug, 117, 137
  behavior disorder, 146
  narcolepsy, 75

175

Lingual obstruction, 144
Lipoidoses, 88
Literature, current, *Epilepsy Abstracts*, vii
Liver damage, 115, 122, 123, 127, 129, 130, 132, 134, 138
Lobectomy, anterior temporal, 58, 59
Lobotomy, frontal, 149
Lymphadenopathy, 123
Lymphoma, 120

M

Macropsia, 40, 64
Malaise, 15, 65
Malaria, 95
Male, ratio in epilepsy, 23, 36, 45
Malignancy, of brain tumor, 104
Malingering, 80–83
Marriage, 153, 154
Masked epilepsy, 63–65
Massive myoclonia, 22, 37
  see also Hypsarhythmia
Maturational process, 8, 9
  see also Age factor
Maximal seizures, 8
  see also Grand mal
Measles, 87, 92, 93
Measles-like rash, with drugs, 120–123
Mebaral
  antiepileptic agent, 117, 131
  dosage, 131
  drug combinations, 131
Medico-legal cases, 45, 96
Mellaril, 138
Memory defects, 56, 57, 59
Ménière's syndrome, 80, 81
Meningioma, 50, 104
Meningitis, 94, 95
Mental retardation, 106–108
  behavior disorder, 78, 146
  birth injury, 106, 108–110
  cerebral palsy, 107, 109, 110
  enuresis, 76
  etiology and seizures, 87, 106
  fourteen and six, 44
  hypsarhythmia, 22, 24, 108
  infectious disease, 92, 93, 106
  marriage, 153
  myoclonic epilepsy, 38

petit mal variant, 32, 108
photically induced seizures, 61
status epilepticus, 106, 107
surgical treatment, 142
trauma, 97
Mephobarbital, *see* Mabaral
Meprobamate
  accessory drug, 139
  behavior disorders, 146
  withdrawal convulsions, 74
Mesantoin
  antiepileptic agents, 117, 122–124
  blood count, 123, 124
  dosage, 124
  drug combinations, 122, 123, 126, 128, 147
  porphyria, 88
  SGOT, 123
  side effects, 123, 124
Metabolic disorders, 21, 24, 87, 88, 90, 113
Methamphetamine hydrochloride, *see* Desoxyn
Metharbital, *see* Gemonil
Methsuximide, *see* Celontin
Methyloxyzolidine dione, *see* Paradione
Methylphenylethyl hydantoin, *see* Mesantoin
Metrazol activation, 18
Microcephaly, 24
Micropsia, 40, 64
Midtemporal focus, and
  age factor, 8, 9, 51
  anterior temporal involvement, 54, 57
  audiogenic seizures, 62
  behavior disturbances, 78
  cardiovascular disease, 102
  cerebral palsy, 111
  fourteen and six, 42
  laterality, 50
  masked epilepsy, 65
  nightmares, 76
  psychomotor variant, maximal, 45
  small sharp spikes, maximal, 18
  symptoms, 52
  trigeminal neuralgia, 71
  tumor, 103
Migration of foci, 52
  see also Age factor